# THE KNOW LEDGE

## DR NIGHAT ARIF

Your guide to female health from menstruation to the menopause

ASTER*

# Contents

**PHASE 3**

# Your Midlife Years

# Introduction

Back in the spring of 2019, I was working at a practice in rural Buckinghamshire as a GP with a special interest in women's health. That area of medicine had always fascinated me, from menstruation through to menopause, and helping people to access the right care and treatment had become my vocation and my passion.

Alongside my GP duties, I began to create social media posts to raise awareness of various topics; the importance of cervical screening, for instance, or the benefits of HRT. I wanted to use my experience as a clinician to empower women with knowledge, to encourage them to get to know their bodies and to dispel the myths that were often perpetuated within the area of women's health. To communicate these important messages in the most effective manner possible, I took great care to use clear language, factual terminology and evidence-based data. Furthermore, as someone with Pakistani heritage, I was keen to reach out to a South Asian audience, so I produced content in Urdu and Punjabi as well as English.

My tweets, TikTok and Instagram posts began to gather momentum and soon caught the attention of the *BBC Breakfast* team. In May 2019, they invited me onto the show to discuss the common symptoms of menopause and my efforts to raise awareness in the ethnic minority community. This appearance by a 30-something, hijab-wearing Muslim woman caused quite a stir, not just because I was talking openly about night sweats and vaginal dryness – considered taboo subjects by many – on a flagship TV programme, but also because GPs who looked like me were rarely seen on TV. The positive feedback I received as a consequence – especially from women of colour – completely blew me away.

More TV appearances followed (including ITV's *This Morning*) and my social media hits skyrocketed. I received thousands of responses from people across the globe who had watched one of my videos, recognized their own symptoms and – armed with new-found information – had checked in with a healthcare professional. As a GP this was music to my ears, of course, but it also highlighted a huge demand for clear, factual and accessible advice. And that, in a nutshell, is what prompted me to grab my laptop and write *The Knowledge*.

I want to share my expertise. I want to start a conversation. I want you to understand your body, to identify any changes and to realize when – and how – to seek help. Ultimately, I want you to look after yourself in the best way possible so you can lead a long, happy and healthy life. You may not find every single answer within these pages – medicine is rarely one-size-fits-all, and no two people experience the same symptoms – but if you spot a nugget of advice that prompts you to pick up the phone to your doctor, or encourages you to perform your first self examination, then this labour of love will have served its purpose.

I have intentionally divided the book into three phases, to reflect the main stages in a woman's life journey: puberty, fertility and menopause. I firmly believe that everyone assigned female at birth, regardless of age, should learn about these distinct phases and the changes they embrace. Indeed, during the writing process I found it helpful to view things from the perspective of my 14-year-old self. I was raised in a traditional, religious Muslim household where women's health matters were hardly discussed, so I had to use other means to learn about things like menstruation and contraception. The teenage 'me' would have undoubtedly appreciated a book like this, as it would have given me a deeper understanding of myself… and a deeper understanding of my mother and grandmother!

And while I want to help women and girls of all ages, I'm just as keen to help their loved ones, too – that's mums, dads, siblings, grandparents and other relatives or care-givers. I particularly want to reach out to fathers, perhaps those who are single, separated or widowed – or in same-sex relationships – who may not have female partners to consult. It's so important that you feel comfortable talking to your daughters about period products, or family planning, and can do so openly and honestly.

Removing the shame and stigma from women's health is an on-going mission of mine and forms a central theme of this book. The embarrassment factor can prove to be fatal, quite literally, if it prevents someone from getting the right care at the right time. Gynaecological cancers claim thousands of lives each year but, by performing self examinations of your breast tissue, vulva and vagina – and having regular smear tests – any changes or anomalies may be spotted early enough for you to obtain successful treatment. We also need to encourage our children and young people to familiarize themselves with their genitals without feeling ashamed. By normalizing these matters – girls checking their vulvas, boys checking their penises – good habits will be formed and infection and disease may be averted. So much of my work as a GP involves this kind of preventative care; it genuinely does save lives.

*The Knowledge* also offers help and advice for individuals who don't fit the mould of what society – and the healthcare system – still deem as 'normal' (although I always question this concept, because in medicine there's no such thing as a 'normal' period, for example, or a 'normal' menopause). I'm very proud of the fact that this book includes guidance for trans people and those with disabilities. These individuals have exactly the same rights to sexual and reproductive healthcare as any other patient, and should receive treatment without discrimination or prejudice. This content may also be useful to fellow clinicians, who should be ensuring their surgeries and consultations are as inclusive and as accessible as possible.

I apply a similar principle to people struggling with infertility or baby loss, whose circumstances should never be overlooked or underplayed. Successful conception, pregnancy and childbirth is still very much part of the common narrative, meaning that those who encounter problems often feel excluded from the conversation.

Many women of colour can feel side-lined, too; institutional racism, combined with systemic misogyny, continues to prevail in the healthcare sector and I still hear appalling stories from women of colour whose symptoms are dismissed and whose pain is invalidated. I'm determined to combat this, and will continue to call for allies to fight our corner and for ambassadors to connect with communities.

And let me be clear: should anyone query why inclusivity, diversity and ally-ship is so important to me, and why it forms such an intrinsic part of my ethos (and this book), I'll always flip it around to ask, 'Well, why shouldn't it be important? And why should the question even need to be asked in the first place?' As far as I'm concerned, the basic principles of medicine are universal. Gold-standard healthcare should be available to all. No one should face bias or exclusion; on the contrary, they should all have a place at the table.

As a member of an ethnic group, and an employee of the UK's National Health Service (NHS), the issue of representation really matters to me. It's a known fact that most promotional healthcare material – leaflets, posters, diagrams and illustrations – does not always feature people of colour. This, quite understandably, can send the wrong signals to people who may already feel excluded from mainstream medicine, and who are therefore less likely to engage with clinicians. I'm doing my utmost to challenge and change this, and am immensely proud of the diverse (and ground-breaking!) illustrations that have been specially created for this book. I only wish they'd existed when I was younger; back then, public health messaging was distinctly white, Western and middle class.

I'm also keen to break down the cultural barriers that prevent women of colour from accessing the care they need. Many of their health issues, including menstruation and menopause, are kept 'under the veil' (not spoken about, in other words), which can have a severe impact on their wellbeing. To these people – and to anybody else who's feeling alone and isolated – I truly hope I can help you to find your voice and start that conversation.

But along with being heard, you also need to feel seen. And as someone who eats, sleeps and breathes clinical medicine, I want you to know that I see you. I see you suffering with endometriosis. I see you living with perimenopause. I see you coping with infertility. I see you struggling with gender identity. I see you simply wanting to be sure that your periods are normal. This book, I hope, will empower you to get the healthcare you deserve and, not only that, will encourage you to spread the word and tell your story. Your knowledge is a gift, to be shared freely with others. I hope this book plays a role in providing a pillar of support on that journey.

Finally, each one of us carries a candle of knowledge. Kindled by wisdom and experience, it brings light, warmth and energy. But we shouldn't keep the candle to ourselves. We should use it to light somebody else's. That way, the flame continues to burn brightly.

With love,

Dr Nighat Arif

Dear body,
thank you for
harbouring me,
making me beautiful,
nourishing me,
making me capable of
remarkable things.
I promise to love and
respect you.

# Female anatomy & self examinations

··········································································

Awareness of your own body is key to good health, so it's vital that you educate yourself about your basic anatomy, both internal and external. On the following pages are diagrams of the internal female reproductive system and breasts, as well as a diagram of the external vulva and pubic area. These should really help as a reference point for many sections of the book that follow.

While much of your internal anatomy won't be visible to you, it is still vital that you have a keen awareness of how areas of your body look and feel – because every body is different, only you can know your own body best. If I had my own way, every woman or person assigned female at birth (AFAB) would examine their breast tissue and genitals on a regular basis from the age of 13. Ideally, by the time you are 18, you should complete all self examinations once a month, in between periods. The more we learn about the way we look, and the way things feel, the more likely we'll be to notice changes and spot anomalies. Flagging up any concerns to your doctor may help them recognize certain symptoms and make early (sometimes life-saving) diagnoses. Pages 16–17 and 21–3 will show you how to undertake these self examinations in detail.

# The female reproductive system

The female reproductive system includes everything involved in creating and carrying a baby, but it is so important to have an awareness of your system at every stage of your life, even if you never intend to have a pregnancy. The system begins at the vulva, the external element that you can see in your self examination (see pages 21–3), then moves into the vagina and then the cervix, which is the opening to the uterus. The uterus is lined with the endometrium and is where, if you are pregnant, the foetus will grow and be supported throughout your pregnancy. If you are not pregnant, then your menstrual cycle runs through a process of thickening the endometrium and then shedding the lining with your period. The ovaries are where an egg (ovum) matures each month, which is then released into the fallopian tube to travel along towards the uterus.

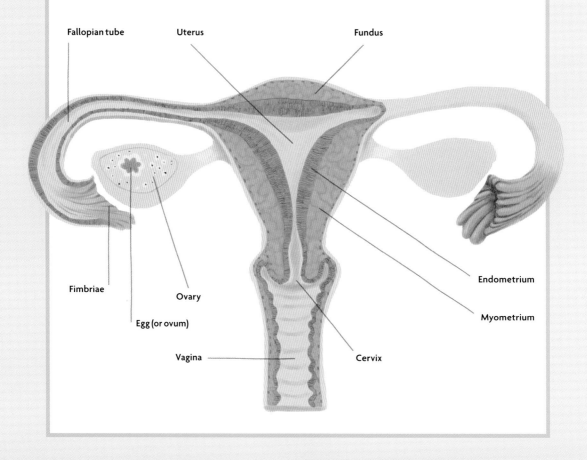

Fallopian tube

Uterus

Fundus

Fimbriae

Ovary

Egg (or ovum)

Vagina

Cervix

Endometrium

Myometrium

# The female reproductive system (side view)

People are frequently surprised by how close the reproductive system is to the lower part of the digestive system, but they are all snugly clustered together within the pelvis. This is particularly important to note during times when your natural levels of the hormone oestrogen drops, as this is the reason why vaginal atrophy (see page 168) can cause infections in the urinary tract. Your bladder and urethra sit just in front of your uterus and labia, while the bowel, rectum and anus sit just behind. Between the lower opening of the vulva and the rectum is an area called the perineum, which can easily split or become sore if the skin becomes dry.

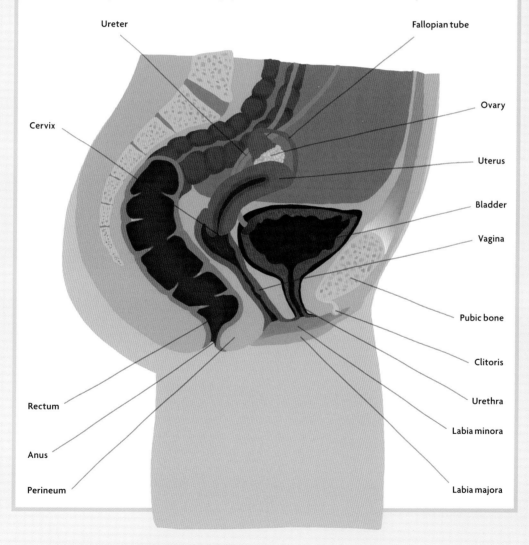

Ureter

Fallopian tube

Cervix

Ovary

Uterus

Bladder

Vagina

Pubic bone

Clitoris

Urethra

Rectum

Labia minora

Anus

Perineum

Labia majora

## The vulva & pubic area

The vulva is the external part of your genitals while the pubic area is that between your legs, above your vulva, where your pubic hair grows. Looking into the vulva you will see that it's formed of the outer labia and inner labia. The clitoral hood sits at the top of the inner labia and covers the clitoris, while the urethral opening (where you urinate from) is just below. The entrance to the vagina sits at the bottom of the inner labia, then the perineum is an area of skin that sits between the openings of the vagina and the anus.

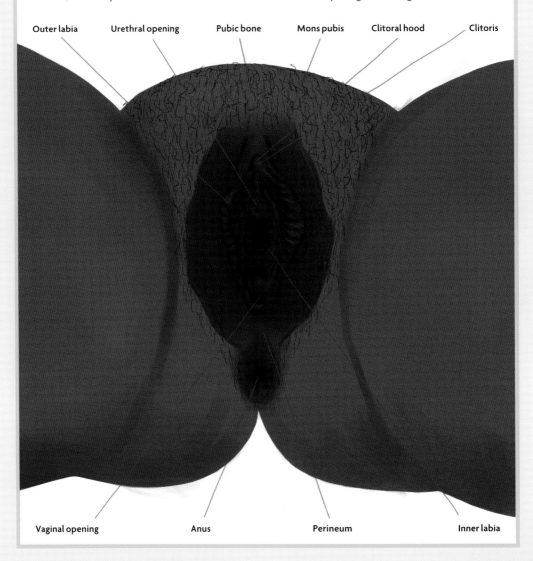

Outer labia    Urethral opening    Pubic bone    Mons pubis    Clitoral hood    Clitoris

Vaginal opening    Anus    Perineum    Inner labia

# The breast

The breasts sit in front of the chest, separated from your ribs by the pectoral muscles. Each breast is formed of several lobules (or alveoli), around 15 to 20 in each breast, that are connected via milk ducts and milk reservoirs to tiny openings in the nipple. The hormonal changes associated with late pregnancy and childbirth will stimulate the alveoli to make milk and the action of a baby suckling at the breast will cause a 'let down', when the milk is released from the alveoli, through the milk ducts and reservoirs out through the nipple openings. The first milk that comes from the breast is a rich, fatty substance called colostrum and then the 'mature' milk will be produced about two days after a baby is born.

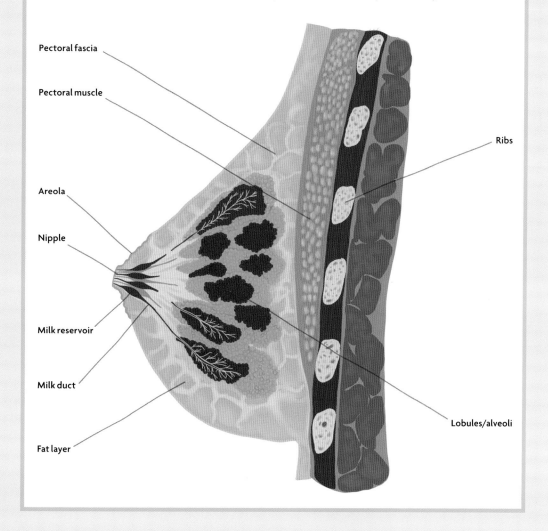

Pectoral fascia

Pectoral muscle

Ribs

Areola

Nipple

Milk reservoir

Milk duct

Lobules/alveoli

Fat layer

# Self examination: Breasts

Thanks to the increased raising of awareness throughout the NHS – and the fabulous work of charities like Breast Cancer Now – more women are examining their breast tissue than ever before. A thorough self examination should take about ten minutes and might just save your life.

## Examining your breasts

I advise my patients to do breast examinations on a monthly basis: on roughly the same date each month, or two weeks before or after your period, if you're menstruating (as fluctuations in oestrogen around your period are likely to cause breast pain and swelling that might mean missing any lumps).

Perform your breast exam wherever it feels comfortable (preferably somewhere nice and quiet, where you won't be disturbed) – perhaps on your bed, or in the bath or shower. I often tell my patients to do it at a particular time of day, which might help to jog their memory and make it a routine, perhaps in front of their bedroom mirror as they're getting dressed for work on a Monday morning. I know some women who ask their partners to have a good feel of their breast tissue – you'd be surprised how many lumps are found by loved ones – and you can always return the favour by assisting with their personal examinations. It's important to point out that those assigned male at birth can get breast cancer too, so it's a good idea for them to check their pecs regularly.

Breast implants can make a self examination more difficult but it is still important. You should be able to gently shift the position of the implant and you can then palpate around the implant to feel the breast tissue around it.

## What to look out for during a breast self examination

- A new lump in the breast or armpit area, which may or may not cause pain.
- Irritation, redness, darkening or flaking of the skin around the breast and nipple area.
- A swelling or thickening in any part of the breast.
- Skin snagging, puckering or dimpling around the nipple area.
- Nipple discharge or blood if not pregnant or nursing.
- A marked and visible change in breast size (it's common for women to have one breast bigger than the other, but watch out for *recent* changes).
- A dull or sharp pain in any area of the breast.

Try to focus and concentrate as you feel your breasts. Don't be half-hearted or absent-minded! Remind yourself that you're feeling for lumps and bumps in the breast tissue and armpit area, and are looking for any changes in the skin or nipple.

If you *do* notice any irregularities during a self examination, try not to panic or assume the worst. Make a note of these changes, however small, and book an appointment to see your doctor as soon as possible, outlining the reasons to the receptionist when you call.

Do not delay matters or tell yourself that you're worrying unnecessarily. The sooner you get seen by a clinician, the better. And – should anything require further investigation – you'll be promptly referred to a specialist.

# How to examine your breasts

Examine your breast tissue monthly, preferably between your periods. Find somewhere you are comfortable, either standing up or lying on your back. Then remove your top and bra. Complete the following steps on both sides.

1 With the pads of four fingers, slowly press around the fleshy breast tissue in a circular motion, moving outwards from the nipple to your rib and armpit areas. Apply pressure that's firm, but comfortable. Feel for any changes to the flesh or skin as outlined opposite.

2 Use your fingers to feel underneath and around the nipple, looking for any changes to the flesh or skin.

3 Use your fingers to feel underneath the armpit, looking for any changes to the flesh or skin.

4 Walk your fingers up your chest towards the neck, feeling as you go, looking for any changes to the flesh or skin.

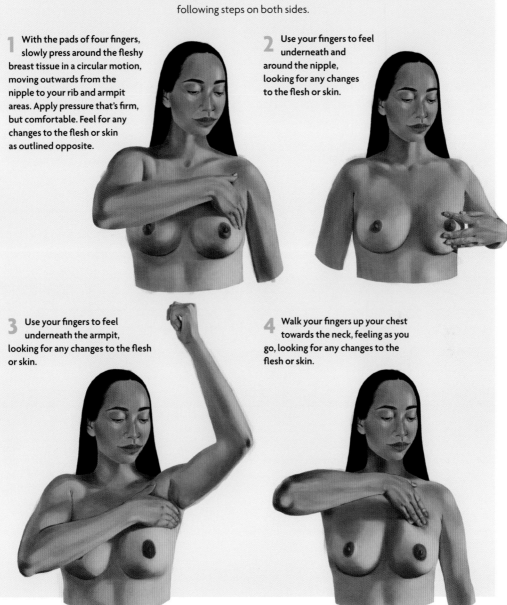

# Wear the correct size bra!

I see so many women in my surgery with chronic breast pain who are clearly wearing the wrong-sized bra. When I was younger, I never received any guidance about the importance of wearing the right bra. I was none the wiser until the age of 23, when a lovely lady in the lingerie department of a local shop introduced me to the joys (and comfort) of wearing a correctly fitted bra!

The easiest way to find your bra size is to visit the lingerie section of your local department store, or a stand-alone lingerie store. The staff there will be specially trained in measuring busts. Many bra-fitters now determine your size on sight, without a tape measure – a real specialist skill! If, however, you don't feel comfortable visiting a store, or can't find the time to, then you can measure yourself at home, and calculate your bra size from there.

## How to measure your bra size

You'll need to take two measurements to determine your bra size: the band measurement and the cup measurement. If possible measure in inches (because that's how bra sizes are calculated), but you can use an online calculator to convert this to centimetres if your tape measure doesn't show inches.

To find the band size, measure all around your ribcage just beneath your breasts. (If the measurement is an odd number then scale up or down to the nearest even number.) This number is your band size. Then measure all around the widest area of your bust, so the tape measure sits firmly but comfortably. Subtracting this measurement from your band size will give your cup size, so less than 1 inch (2.5cm) = AA, 1 inch (2.5cm) = A, 2 inches (5cm) = B, 3 inches (7.5cm) = C, 4 inches (10cm) = D, 5 inches (12.7cm) = DD, 6 inches (15.2cm) = E, 7 inches (17.8cm) = F, 8 inches (20.3cm) = FF,

9 inches (22.9cm) = G, 10 inches (25.4cm) = GG, 11 inches (27.9cm) = H. Sizes beyond H are usually available from specialist retailers.

## What to look for in a well-fitting bra

- It should be snug when on the loosest hook.
- The shoulder strap should sit comfortably to prevent shoulder pain.
- The cups should be flush with your bust.
- The centre wire or fabric should sit flat against the chest wall; if it pulls away the cup is not deep enough, and if it wobbles the cup is too deep.
- At the sides, the bra wire or fabric should sit under the breast along the ribs; if it sits on the breast tissue, the cup is too small, and if the side wire is too big it will dig into the underarm area.

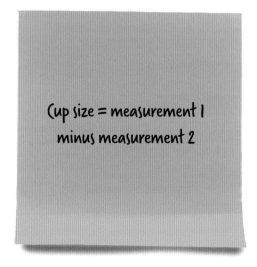

Cup size = measurement 1 minus measurement 2

## How to measure your bra size

Find somewhere you can measure yourself comfortably without being distracted, then either measure over a soft (non-padded) bra – whichever bra you currently find most comfortable to wear – or against your bare breasts.

**1** Measure the circumference around the fullest part of your breasts (shown by the solid line below). The tape measure should have a little give in this measurement.

**2** Measure the circumference around your ribcage beneath your breasts (shown by the dotted line below). The tape measure should be very snug, but still comfortable for this measurement.

**3** Calculate your bra size using the formula opposite.

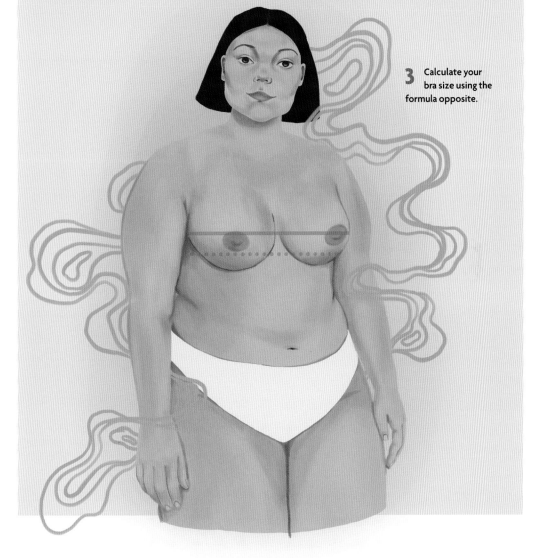

Remember: no two vulvas look the same, each is completely unique. And no one should know your vulva and vagina better than you.

So why not grab a mirror and get started?

# Self examination: Vulva & pubic area

Whilst breast self examinations have become commonplace – and saved countless lives – there is still a huge lack of awareness around genital self examinations. This simply has to change if we are going to reduce the incidence of vaginal and vulval cancers, so it is vital you familiarize yourself with your vulva and pubic area.

## Examining your vulva & pubic area

Vulval and vaginal cancers are rare but frequently missed or misdiagnosed (see page 150). They can occur in women of any age, more often among those who are long-term smokers or who have a family history of melanoma (a type of skin cancer). There are 1,400 new cases of vulval cancer each year in the UK and five every week of vaginal cancer. While they are awful diseases, if picked up early, then the prognosis is encouraging. Self examination is key and, as per usual, this is a euphemism-free zone, so no talk of foo-foos or front bottoms whatsoever!

Not to be confused with the vagina, the vulva is another name for your external genitals, namely the labia majora (outer lips), the labia minora (inner lips) and the clitoris. Speaking as a doctor who has examined thousands of women, I can assure you that no two vulvas look alike. Becoming familiar with the way your vulva looks and feels is very, very important.

If we're going to raise awareness about vulval examinations, however, we first have to remove the stigma and take away the sexualization of women's bodies in today's society. Examining and touching your vulva for health purposes isn't remotely pornographic – it's a sensible thing to do, not a sexual thing to do – and we need the men in our lives to respect and support us in this regard.

We also need to reach the stage where we can encourage our children to regularly examine their genitals without embarrassment. By normalizing things – girls checking their vulvas every week, boys checking their penises and testicles – good habits will be formed and infections and diseases may be recognized and treated at an early stage.

A vulval examination should ideally take place monthly: on roughly the same date each month, similarly to a breast examination (I often encourage my patients to get into the routine of doing the examinations one after another). You'll need some privacy – and won't want interruptions, of course – so perhaps choose a locked bathroom or bedroom, preferably with some natural light. Find yourself a small hand-held mirror, and set aside ten minutes or so.

## What to look out for during a vulva & pubic region self examination

* Any lumps, bumps, spots or sores that could indicate infection, disease or other conditions.
* Any changes to the colour or size of different areas from one examination to the next.
* Any bad-smelling discharge (though some discharge is normal, and the amount will depend on what point you are at in your menstrual cycle). If your discharge has a bad smell or is an unusual colour (see page 70), it could indicate an infection.

# How to examine your vulva & pubic region

Examine your vulva monthly, preferably between your menstrual periods, if you have them. Before you begin, wash your hands with soap and water, then grab a hand-held mirror and find somewhere with enough space to sit, squat or lie down, on the floor or on a chair, and sufficient light for you to see well, where you won't be interrupted for ten minutes.

**1** Open your legs and check the area where your pubic hair grows. Feel around with your fingers and position your mirror to check for moles, bumps, spots, warts, ulcers, lesions, rashes or white patches. Make a mental note of anything that looks new or feels different. Examine the fleshy area from top to bottom.

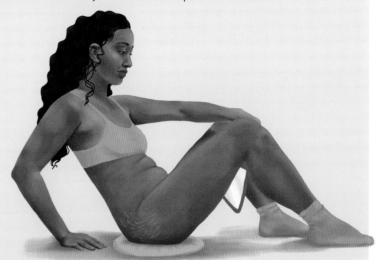

**2** Next, find your clitoris – at the top of the vulva, the fold of skin where the inner labia meet – and look for any bumps, growths or discolouration.

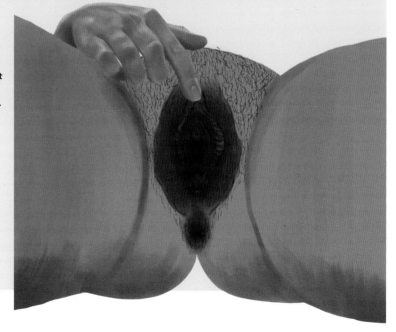

**3** Check your labia majora – the outer lips – and, again, feel for any bumps, spots, lesions or rashes.

**4** Check your labia minora – the inner lips – and, again, feel for any bumps, spots, lesions or rashes.

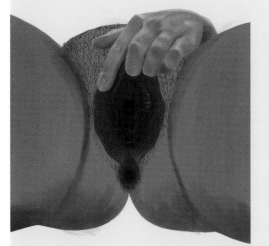

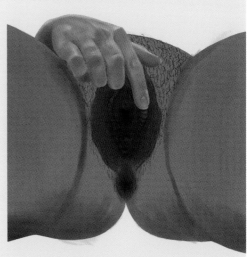

**5** Prop the mirror in front of you and use one hand to gently hold open your labia minora, to see into your vagina. Check your vagina for any bumps, spots, lesions or rashes. You may see what looks like 'rings' going around the vaginal wall – this is called mucosal tissue and is completely normal.

**6** Finally, check your perineum (the area located between the entrance to the vagina and the anus) for any lumps, bumps or anomalies. When you have finished, wash your hands again. Make a note of any changes detected and, if you're at all worried about any anomalies, don't hesitate to consult your doctor for a professional examination.

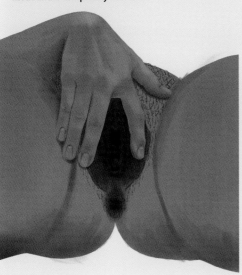

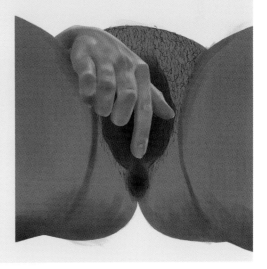

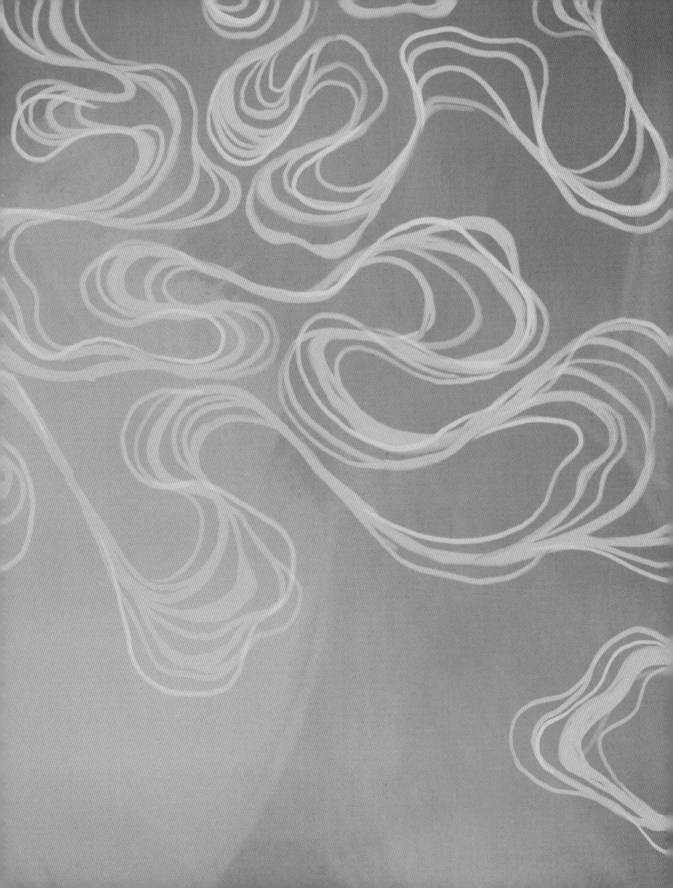

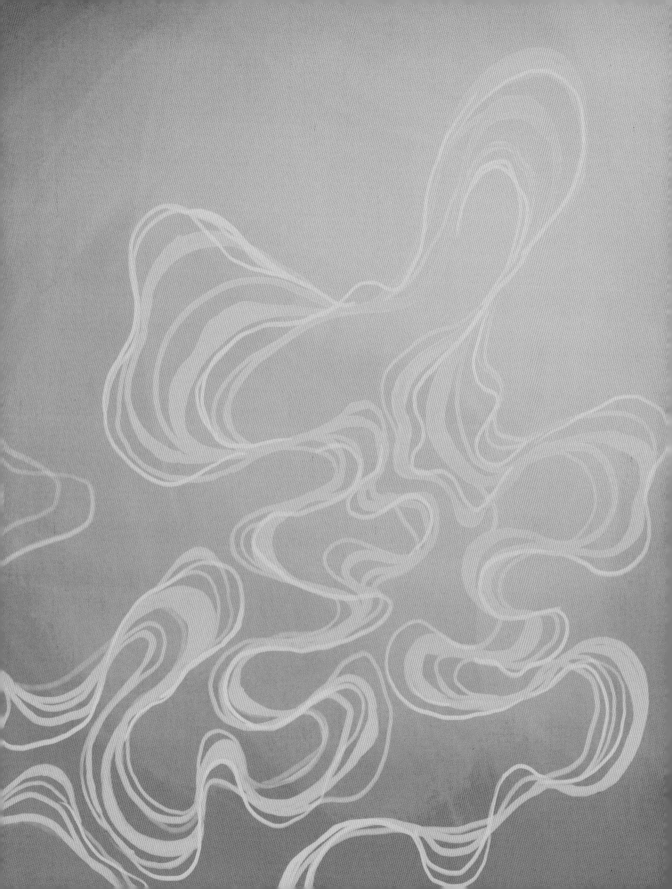

# Fair healthcare access for all

..........................................

I feel strongly that everybody – whatever their creed, colour, background, ability or gender expression – should have equal access to healthcare when they visit my surgery or any other service in the healthcare system.

However, this is still not the case for many people trying to access healthcare and advice. Patients can be discriminated against for many reasons and access to fair healthcare for ethnic minorities, those who are disabled and the LGBTQ+ community is woefully below the ideal standards. In order to counterbalance this, and to ensure that such disparity and discrimination is eradicated, we need allies to help fight our corner, and ambassadors to try to connect with our communities.

# Ethnic minorities

Institutional racism and systemic misogyny continue to prevail in healthcare, to the detriment of ethnic minority women. The health issues of women of colour are often dismissed by clinicians or their own community, and their pain is downplayed and invalidated.

In some ethnic minority communities, when someone is unwell they're more likely to have a mindset of 'I will be cured if I pray hard enough' or 'this is a test of my faith'. This can lead to a reticence to address any symptoms with a doctor, and the shame and stigma will persist. Women are also less likely to discuss women's health matters with others in their community – whether that's talking about examining themselves, or about a lump they've found – and this inhibits vital information sharing. It's really important for us to recognize this issue within ethnic minority communities, and to realize that more health advocates are needed in situ to raise awareness and strengthen messages.

I'm all too aware that, among Black and Asian ethnic minorities, there's still a lot of shame and stigma around breast examinations, for example. Within some parts of society – particularly faith-based communities – breasts are highly sexualized, prompting the mindset that they're something to keep hidden. This often deters women from checking their breasts at home, or having them examined by a doctor. Whatever their symptoms, ethnic minority women are also more likely to wait for an appointment with a female doctor which, due to sheer demand, can lead to a delay. If you have an immediate health concern you may be seen much quicker by a male doctor, who will be more than happy to offer you a chaperone, or let a friend of family member accompany you.

When you make a medical appointment, don't be afraid to state your preferences:

- If you feel uncomfortable being seen by a doctor of a particular gender, you may state your preference to the receptionist.
- Ask to bring someone with you to your appointment (a friend or family member) or, alternatively, you can put in an advance request for the surgery to provide a chaperone; this might be another health professional.

All doctor's surgeries will offer you a chaperone during an appointment if you prefer, or will let you take a friend or family member with you.

If English isn't your first language, and none of the doctors happen to speak your first language, you can ask the receptionist to book an interpreter for you or, if you prefer, bring someone to the appointment who can translate for you.

### Removing barriers

Language can be a significant obstacle for women whose mother tongue is Urdu or Punjabi, for example, and who are unable to see a doctor who speaks it. Talking about menopause or other women's health issues can be embarrassing enough for these patients, but saying 'my night sweats soak my sheets' or 'sex with my husband is really painful' via a family chaperone or an interpreter can be problematic. In order to address these issues, not only do we need a more ethnically diverse workforce in the healthcare sector, we also need Western-trained doctors (myself included) to recognize these cultural barriers.

A lack of understanding about women's health can prevent ethnic minority women from accessing the care they need. It's become a personal mission of mine to target more evidence-based information at these hard-to-reach communities, and I regularly post short videos and longer-form interviews and Q&As on social media. Most of my posts on TikTok, Twitter and Instagram are spoken or subtitled in Urdu and Punjabi, as I've realized that many women in those communities will respond much better to verbal rather than written information (illiteracy levels are particularly high among first-generation South Asian female migrants). My social media feeds share the same handle – @DrNighatArif – so please feel free to watch and share.

> If English isn't your first language, you can ask for a translator if necessary (although you may have to be quite insistent).

### Improving representation

Most healthcare-related promotional material – including many leaflets, posters and illustrations – does not feature people of colour. This can send the wrong message to ethnic minorities who feel excluded from mainstream medicine and are less likely to engage with healthcare professionals. I'm doing my utmost to try to change this. In 2019 I worked with the Pausitivity campaign group to produce a #KnowYourMenopause poster in Urdu, specifically aimed at connecting with midlife women in South Asian communities. Being the first of its kind, the poster had a massive impact when it was distributed to doctors' surgeries and community centres across the UK. A poster was also produced in Welsh, too.

Over the last few years I've also had the privilege of appearing on TV programmes including *BBC Breakfast* and ITV's *This Morning* to discuss medical matters, often from a women's health perspective, which range from hot flushes to vaginal dryness. The response from my South Asian sisters has been overwhelmingly positive. They appreciate watching someone on TV who speaks for them and looks like them; let's be honest, there aren't many Muslim women wearing pink hijabs on national TV! There's no doubt about it...representation matters.

# 8.9%
## of residents of England and Wales did not have English as their main language in 2021

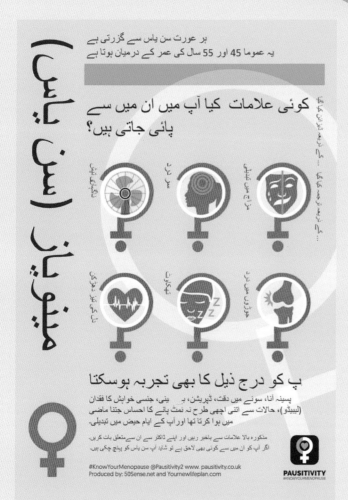

Left: My 2019 collaboration with Pausitivity, which produced posters in Urdu to raise awareness of menopause symptoms in the South Asian community. The Pausitivity team also produced a Welsh-language poster to increase awareness in Welsh-speaking communities. Posters reproduced with thanks to Elizabeth Carr-Ellis and the Pausitivity team.

# Women's health & disability

In order to reduce barriers to healthcare, doctors should make their surgeries and consultations as accessible as possible, and we should be acting as ambassadors and allies for all patients.

A 2021 article entitled 'Barriers in access to healthcare for women with disabilities' in the *BMC Women's Health* journal stated that 'women with disabilities (WWD) are more likely to have unmet healthcare needs than women without disabilities'. This statement was corroborated by the following findings outlined by the Sisters of Frida organization, a collective of disabled women:

- Disabled women have limited access to prenatal care and reproductive health services.
- Most maternity care does not meet the needs of disabled women.
- Disabled, older, asylum-seeking and Traveller women face obstacles in accessing healthcare.

In my own practice, I strive to ensure that any of my patients with physical disabilities receive the same healthcare as my able-bodied patients, and I will consider certain practicalities, such as adapting the way I fit a wheelchair user with a coil, or discussing which period products might suit their circumstances. I'll always outline the risks and benefits to an individual so they are in total control of their decision; empowering my patients is what I'm here for! If a patient is visually impaired, I'll often record voice notes, instead of writing things down or printing things out.

I also tend to use audio-based instructions for anyone who has difficulties with reading: summarizing their contraceptive options via voice notes on their phone, for instance, will always optimize healthcare for these people more than a factsheet or website. Patients with hearing loss are welcome to attend my consultations with a British Sign Language (BSL) interpreter. This is often a friend or family member but outside of this, the options are sadly limited. (A free remote interpreting service – BSL Health Access – was set up in 2020 to enable deaf people to access phone consultations but, at the time of writing, is sadly no longer funded.) Clarity of communication is vitally important when you're discussing life-changing decisions, and I hope this barrier will be removed soon.

Consultations can also be complex if I'm seeing a patient with a cognitive impairment, perhaps associated with a condition like Down's syndrome or Huntington's disease, or with neurodiverse conditions. In these instances, the way in which I communicate their healthcare options, and the way I obtain medical consent, often has to be adjusted. While I'll endeavour to involve the patient as much as possible, if they are unable to make cognitive decisions about fertility or contraception, for example, I may choose to consult with the person who has the patient's best interests at heart and who can make a decision on their behalf, often a parent, sibling or guardian.

These are just some ideas for how the healthcare system can work for all, and I hope these ideas will empower you to request the adjustments *you* may need to get the best healthcare for you and your family, too.

Become your
own advocate.
Get informed,
do your research,
become empowered
and DO NOT accept
discriminatory
behaviour.

# Rights for trans patients (& advice for their doctors)

Fear and apprehension can often deter trans people from seeing their doctor.
This is a heart-breaking situation that can have potentially harmful consequences.

The 2018 Stonewall *LGBT in Britain Health Report* agreed that, while there are 'committed individuals and organizations doing outstanding work' in the NHS and beyond, it is also true that 'instances of discrimination, hostility and unfair treatment in healthcare services are still commonplace'. Indeed, three in five trans people (62 per cent) said they'd experienced a lack of understanding of specific trans health needs by healthcare staff.

In 2021, the TransActual organization conducted their Trans Lives survey, a cross-sectional study that recorded the experiences of trans people, including those of colour and those with disabilities. Their findings were truly depressing. Fourteen per cent of respondents had been refused medical care on at least one occasion, on account of being trans. Fifty-seven per cent of trans people – that's more than half – said they had avoided going to the doctor when unwell. Fifty-three per cent of trans people of colour experienced racism while accessing trans-specific healthcare services, and 60 per cent of disabled respondents reported suffering ableism in similar circumstances.

So how can the GP experience be improved for trans patients? Luckily, significant steps are possible to overcome those barriers and optimize their healthcare and the majority of healthcare professionals are inclusive and supportive of such adaptations and changes. The following advice, I hope, will be helpful to both patients *and* clinicians.

### Changing your name & gender details

Any patient can change their name and gender on their doctor's medical records, and this can be done as an informal decision for those under the age of 16 (before they can legally change their name via deed poll). An individual can also state their preferred pronouns, whether it's he/him, she/her or they/them, for example. Surgeries should have a specific form for this purpose, which can usually be provided by the admin team. Your details will be updated on the practice IT network, and will appear on your doctor's computer screen, so there should be no need to 'explain' yourself at an appointment, which can be upsetting. More recently I've got into the habit of asking all my patients to confirm their preferred pronouns; I think it's quite an empowering thing to do.

### Surgery trans policy

Ideally, your surgery will have a trans health policy and, even better, a practitioner who has a specialist interest in trans healthcare who will be best placed to understand your emotional and physical needs.

For those doctors who feel their knowledge is lacking in this area – or needs updating – there are many opportunities for further learning and continuous professional development and I'd like to encourage all doctors (and people!) to be aware of trans issues and how they can affect the individuals concerned.

### Routine cancer screening

When a trans person changes their gender details, they are often issued with a new NHS number. It's really important to obtain confirmation from the doctor's surgery that your data has been migrated successfully so that you'll continue to receive invites for national cancer screening programmes.

Trans men, trans women and non-binary people aged 50-plus should receive an invite for a mammogram if they have breast tissue (due to either naturally occurring oestrogen or oestrogen hormone replacement). A trans man with a uterus will need to attend a cervical smear test every three years between the ages of 25 and 49, and every five years after that until they are 65.

Trans people who've changed their gender marker may not necessarily receive automatic call and recall invites for the relevant cancer screenings so please check that you've not been missed off any lists by flagging this with your healthcare provider. Ideally, there should be a member of staff with sole responsibility for keeping track of the trans patients in the recall system; my own practice has a nurse dedicated to that very task.

### Gender identity clinic referral

I hear many cases of trans people being met with ignorance, even hostility, when they've requested

> It's vital that trans people don't miss out on cancer screening. Double-check with your doctor that you're in the system.

a referral to a gender identity, or gender dysphoria clinic (GDC), perhaps to access gender-specific counselling, medical or surgical affirming therapy, or hormone therapy. This situation requires specialist care, and patients should expect to be treated with dignity and respect before being signposted accordingly (see page 92 for referral options). There is also plenty of valuable guidance for doctors on the General Medical Council website, including shared care agreements and bridging prescriptions.

### Shared care agreements

Some adult trans people (those over the age of 18) choose to access private healthcare for their hormone therapy – often because the waiting list for NHS clinics is so long (often years rather than months). I advise anyone doing this to diligently keep notes of your treatment as, by pursuing the private route, you are in effect becoming your own care-giver (you'll have to monitor your own blood hormone levels, for example).

You can, however, ask your GP to draw up a 'shared-care agreement' that allows an exchange of information between your private clinic and your doctor's surgery. Having these notes to hand will enable your GP to help with any issues associated with your hormone therapy, such as disrupted menstruation, clitoral growth, increased libido, increased facial and body hair (for trans men); or reduced facial and body hair, lower libido, decreased sexual function and genital shrinkage (for trans women).

## Bridging prescriptions

In certain circumstances, adult trans patients who are waiting for treatment at a gender identity clinic can benefit from 'bridging' prescriptions. General Medical Council guidance currently allows GPs (preferably in collaboration with the gender identity clinic) to prescribe hormone treatment to patients who are suffering physically and/or psychologically as they wait for an appointment. In normal circumstances – outside of the bridging prescription remit – GPs are not usually expected to prescribe hormones to trans people unless they have the expertise and knowledge required.

As this has no impact on NHS budgets – hormones are relatively cheap, after all – many clinicians see this as discriminatory. My fellow GP, Dr Kamilla Kamaruddin, is a passionate advocate for trans health and is among those who find this situation problematic. When we last caught up she questioned the fact that GPs could give hormone treatment to cisgender males who had hypogonadism (a condition that can cause erectile dysfunction), the safety profile for which is similar to prescribing testosterone treatment to trans-masculine people. GPs could

also prescribe gonadotropin-releasing hormones to cisgender male patients with prostate cancer, and to cisgender females with endometriosis, but some GPs were reluctant to prescribe hormones to trans patients under a shared-care prescribing agreement with the GDC.

## Complaints procedure

Each surgery has a complaints procedure. If you experience any form of intolerance or discrimination from a doctor, or a member of surgery staff, or if your GP has done nothing to help you, you should report it. You can either register a complaint with your practice manager or contact your local health authority (this advice applies to patients across the board, of course). You are also entitled to request to see a different doctor within your practice, and you can switch your surgery without having to provide a reason. Your local LGBTQ+ group may be able to suggest a more suitable alternative.

When people gain useful knowledge and information about their health issues, they'll go around sprinkling it like confetti...

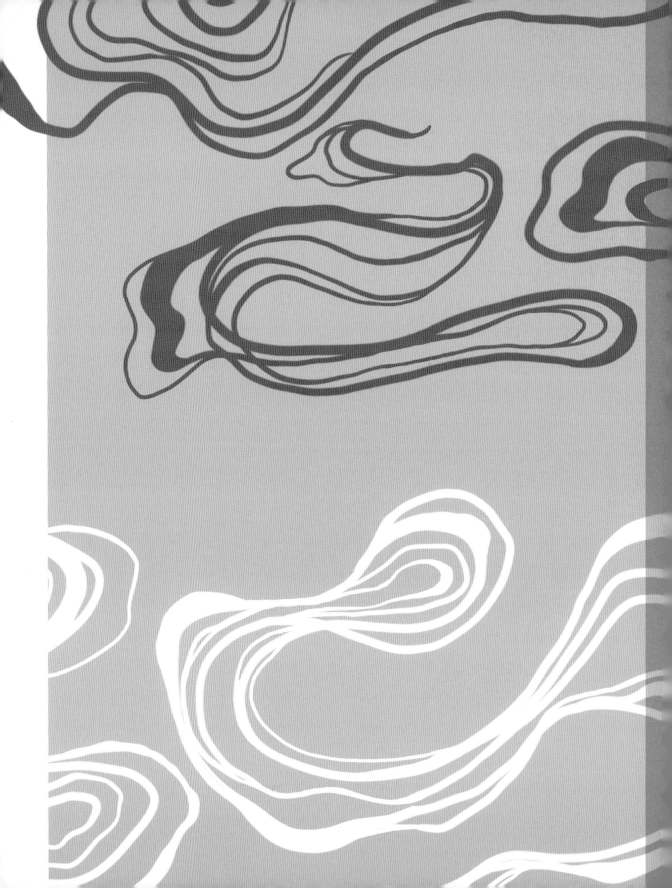

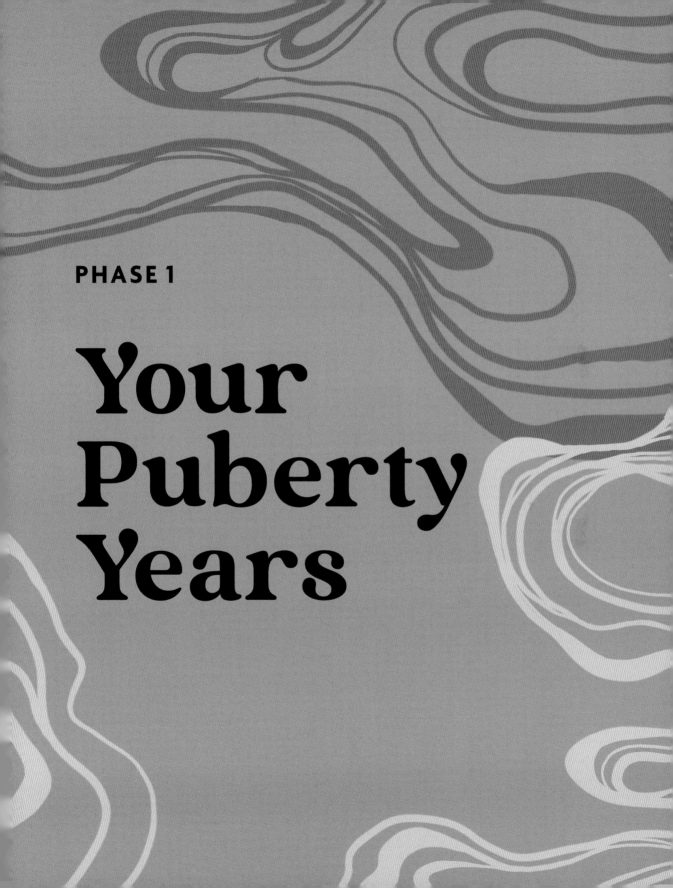

# Your Puberty Years

# Your puberty years: introduction

Girls reach puberty as early as age nine or as late as seventeen, and for many it can be an uncomfortable and disconcerting time. Alongside all the changes that the body undergoes, there's a whole host of emotions and mental health considerations that can make young women feel like they're on a rollercoaster at times. If this is you right now, then I want to take this opportunity to congratulate you on starting this new phase of life. You are becoming more grown up and independent.

I know this stage can feel overwhelming, but I believe that arming yourself with the knowledge of what your body is going through, what to expect (and the huge variations of 'normal' that are possible) and when you should seek additional advice is a really important part of growing up. In this section, I'll talk you through the changes your body will undergo during puberty, as well as the practicalities of dealing with your period and contraception, for when you are ready. In addition, I'll cover issues, both mental and physical, that can arise during your monthly cycle, as well as possible infections and sexually transmitted diseases (STDs), and how they are treated.

# Advice for parents & carers

While I'm very keen for this book to help women and girls understand their bodies, I'm just as keen to inform and educate their loved ones (so that means mums, dads, siblings, grandparents or any other carers or relatives).

I'm especially keen to inform single fathers, or those in same-sex relationships, who don't have a female partner with whom to discuss women's health issues. It's so important that you are able to discuss your daughter's health with her openly.

For starters, parents and carers need to learn to use proper anatomical terms for female genitalia instead of resorting to silly euphemisms. It's a real bugbear of mine. Talking about 'tuppences', 'foo-foos' and 'front bottoms' is not helpful to anyone, and can be really confusing and misleading for a young child (and pretty cringe-worthy for an older child). If we, as the grown-ups in the room, are going to have sensible and practical conversations with our young people about periods and puberty, we need to rid ourselves of the mindset that using anatomical terms is somehow vulgar and inappropriate. It really isn't; in fact, I'd say the opposite is true. So I urge all parents and carers to ditch the daft nicknames and get into the habit of talking about vulvas and vaginas with your children, from their toddler years to their teenage years. Perhaps refer to the illustrations on pages 12–15 as a guide to using the correct genital terminology.

Educating boys about all aspects of women's health is an incredibly important part of their upbringing, in my view. Most will live with women who menstruate or are going through perimenopause, such as their mum, sister or grandmother, yet the subject of women's health is rarely discussed. The boys and men in the household can only benefit from factual information to help them understand these natural bodily functions.

For instance, if you're a parent and your four-year-old spots a tampon in the bathroom and asks what it is, don't just pretend you haven't heard and change the subject. Be honest with him. Use clear and simple language. You could perhaps say, 'Women bleed a little from their vaginas every month. It's called a period. It isn't because they've hurt themselves, it's how their body gets ready in case it needs to make a baby. This is called a tampon. It catches the blood so it doesn't go onto their underwear.' I'm a huge fan of plain and honest speaking!

# Physical changes during puberty

Puberty is a time of significant change: your emotions will be in flux and your body will undergo significant changes. But it is an exciting time as you change from being a child to preparing for adulthood!

Each person experiences the physical changes of puberty at a different rate and there's no specific order, so don't worry if your friend has developed breasts but you haven't. Your time will come! Here are some details of what will change:

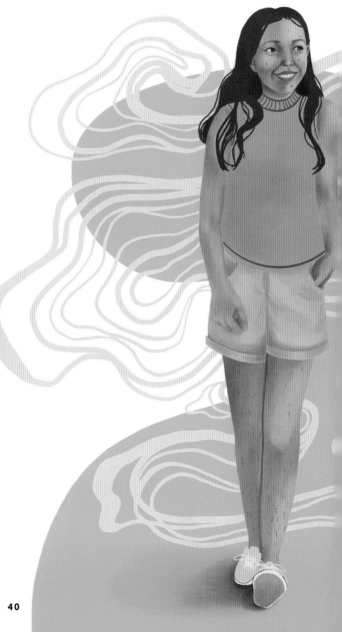

- **Breasts** will develop and grow, and not always at the same rate as one another, so it is completely normal to have one breast bigger than the other. Developing breasts can feel quite tender. As your breasts start to develop it's a good idea to get fitted for a comfortable bra or support top. See pages 18–19 for more details.
- **Height** can increase suddenly as you experience growth spurts during puberty, or you may grow more gradually than your peers.
- **Bodyshape** can become more rounded, especially around the waist, hips and legs.
- **Hair** will develop in your armpits and pubic region, and the rest of your body hair (on your arms and legs in particular) may become thicker.
- **Sweat** increases in volume through puberty and it might be the first time you notice yourself sweating. This can cause body odour so keeping clean and fresh is important.
- **Vaginal discharge** is a thin, clear or whiteish fluid that you may notice in your knickers. This is a natural secretion and helps to keep your vagina healthy and prevents infection.

◆ **Skin** can feel dryer or oiler as hormone levels fluctuate. You may experience outbreaks of spots either around your period or through the month. Acne is a more serious and persistent outbreak of spots that can last beyond puberty. Seek help from your doctor if you would like to explore ways to control spots and acne.

◆ **Periods** are a sign that your uterus is preparing for reproduction (although it may be decades before you decide to have children, if you ever do!). They result in a monthly bleed and there are a range of period products that you can choose to use during this time (see pages 48–51).

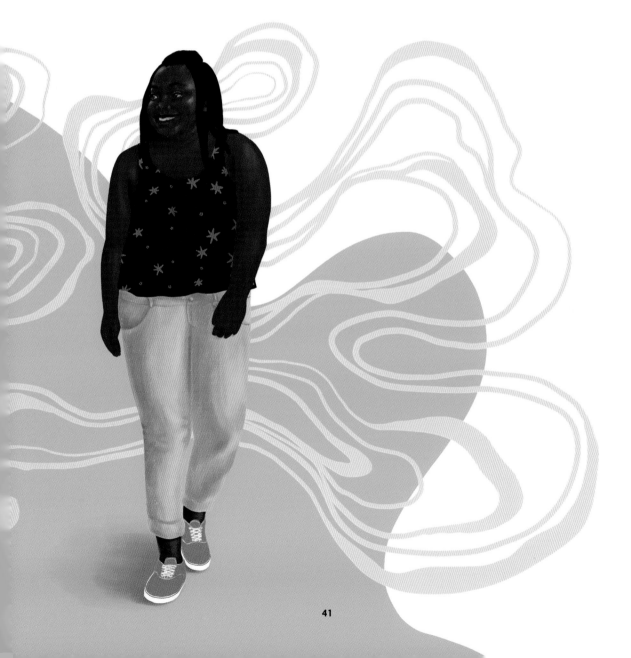

# Periods

Did you know that women, on average, have 500 periods in their lifetime? That's around 12 per year for up to 40 years. However, despite being a normal and natural part of life, periods remain a taboo subject. Many women and girls still don't feel able to speak openly about them, particularly when they have menstrual health problems such as severe pain, heavy bleeding and irregular cycles. According to a survey by Plan International UK, over half of girls in the UK have missed a day or part of a day of schooling due to their period, and around one in three women suffer from heavy menstrual bleeding that can significantly impact their daily life.

We shouldn't be made to feel embarrassed about our periods. This shame and stigma – along with a lack of awareness and education – not only harms women and girls, but also creates barriers to them seeking help. In order to change this, we all need to have more open and honest conversations about menstrual health.

## The phases of your period

Your period is part of the rhythmic change of your reproductive system that is controlled by four hormones: oestrogen, progesterone, follicle stimulating hormone (FSH) and luteinizing hormone (LH). Every 28 days (on average), these hormones cleverly trigger the growth of follicles (fluid-filled sacs containing eggs in the ovaries) and prompt the release of an egg, as well as the growth and shedding of the uterus lining (the endometrium).

If an egg is not fertilized, the endometrial lining – a highly vascular tissue – comes out of the cervix and through the vagina, causing what is commonly known as a period (or menstruation). The first full day of bleeding is counted as day 1 of your menstrual cycle. This cycle comprises three separate phases, based on a 28-day cycle.

### Follicular phase (days 4–14)

The oestrogen hormone triggers the release of the luteinizing hormone (LH) which, at the end of the follicular phase, causes a mature egg to be released from the ovaries into the fallopian tubes (ovulation). You can get pregnant during this time so be aware that sperm can live inside your vagina for several days following unprotected sex.

### Ovulation phase (day 14)

You can usually tell you're ovulating (releasing an egg) by a rise in your body temperature. You may notice your vaginal discharge becoming thicker, too, with a consistency similar to raw egg white. Ovulation usually happens mid-way through your cycle – around day 14 – and lasts around 24 hours. At the time of ovulation, some women can experience spotting (light traces of blood), but many others don't.

### Luteal phase (days 15 onwards)

In this stage, the follicle that released its egg changes into a corpus luteum (a normal clump of cells inside your ovary that forms during each period). This happens immediately after the egg leaves the ovary at ovulation. The corpus luteum releases oestrogen and progesterone. Both these hormones are associated with premenstrual syndrome (PMS, see page 63) which can cause symptoms such as bloating, fatigue, irritability and tearfulness.

If your egg is fertilized in this phase, the progesterone hormone will support early pregnancy. But if it's not fertilized, the corpus luteum will begin to break down, usually about 9–11 days after ovulation. This results in a drop in oestrogen and progesterone levels, which ultimately causes menstruation. The lining of the uterus (the endometrium) secretes chemicals that will either help an early pregnancy or break down the lining – this phase can also be known as the secretory phase.

## Starting your periods

Typically, you will begin your periods about two years after your breasts start developing and, on average, about two years after you notice a white vaginal discharge. Most girls will have their first period around the age of 12, but it does vary from person to person. Some girls can start menstruating when they're just eight or nine, and others can experience their first period at 14 or 15 (both of these scenarios are quite normal). However, if you or a child in your care begin menstruating at seven or eight – something known as 'precocious puberty' – then a visit to the doctor is in order. You should also visit your doctor if you haven't had a period by the age of 16.

**13% of UK schoolgirls miss a day of school** every month due to their period

**EGG → FERTILIZED = PREGNANCY**

. . . . . . . . . . . . . . . . . . . . . . . .

**EGG NOT FERTILIZED → BREAKDOWN OF THE LINING OF THE UTERUS = BLEEDING**

# Endometrial lining & follicle development during your cycle

The endometrial lining breaks down from day 1 of your cycle and is expelled through the vagina. Once shed, the endometrium will thicken through the follicular phase, ovulation and the early luteal phase. At the same time one follicle in one ovary will mature until an egg is ready for release (ovulation), then the egg travels down the fallopian tube and into the uterus. The empty follicle will then close. If the released egg is fertilized then it will attempt to embed in the thickened endometrial lining of the uterus.

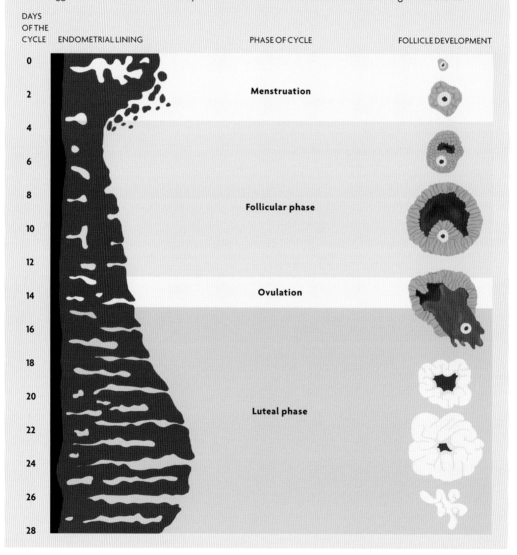

DAYS OF THE CYCLE

ENDOMETRIAL LINING

PHASE OF CYCLE

FOLLICLE DEVELOPMENT

Menstruation

Follicular phase

Ovulation

Luteal phase

## What to expect from your period

In real life there is no such thing as a normal, average period. Everyone is different, with a menstrual cycle and bleeding pattern that are totally unique to them.

### Period length

The length of a period differs from person to person. It usually lasts between five and six days, but can be as short as two to four days, or as long as eight to twelve days. Ideally, though, you need to view your menstrual cycle holistically, instead of just focusing on the days you bleed.

Understanding each different phase will help you to pinpoint the ups and downs of your mood and activity, and to manage your life and routines more effectively.

It's perfectly fine to ask yourself the following questions:

When is the best part of my cycle to make a serious decision?

Which days would be more suitable for me to train hard in the gym?

Which weekend am I more likely to feel confident and outgoing?

Which weekend am I more likely to feel irritable and antisocial?

# FACT:
## a 'normal' period doesn't exist; we all have different cycles

Familiarizing yourself with your menstrual cycle, from start to finish, can be a really useful way to identify your physical and emotional peaks and troughs.

### Period regularity

Most medical text books will state the average menstrual cycle as being 28 days but, from my clinical experience, anything between 21 and 40 days is quite normal if it follows a regular pattern. However, girls who have just started their periods can have very irregular cycles at first – it takes a while for the body to settle into a routine – but if this continues for 12 to 24 months, please do book an appointment to see your doctor.

A woman's menstrual cycle may become irregular for a variety of reasons. Certain conditions can cause the cycle to change – such as fibroids (see page 141), endometriosis (see page 136) and polycystic ovary syndrome (PCOS, see page 130) – and periods may become quite erratic up to eight years before a woman reaches menopause and they stop.

Diet and stress can also have an impact on your menstrual cycle. Sudden or excessive weight loss can cause your periods to become irregular or stop altogether, because the body isn't healthy enough to support a pregnancy. If you have excessive weight gain, the fat cells in your body may produce an increased amount of oestrogen hormone, which can cause periods to become irregular or stop entirely. When we feel stressed, anxious or worried, our body goes into fight-or-flight mode due to a rush of adrenaline and increased cortisol (a steroid hormone). This in turn affects the hormones that trigger ovulation, which can cause disruption to your menstrual cycle. Stress can prompt an early period, irregular periods, late periods or can stop your periods altogether – sometimes for several months.

### Period colour & consistency

The colour of your menstrual blood will change as your period progresses; you might notice that it's brownish at the beginning and end of your bleed, and bright red in the middle.

The consistency and texture of your discharge will also vary, from thin and watery on day 1, perhaps, to thick and sticky on day 3.

Flow and volume will change, too; you may only require a 'regular' pad or tampon in the early stages of your period when your flow is light, but may need to increase it to 'super' as your flow becomes heavier. Remember, these changes are all unique to each unique person.

## The changes to your flow

The volume, colour and texture of menstrual blood will change over your period. Often it will appear a little lumpy and darker at the start (as small clots from the endometrium lining fall away), turning more uniform and bright red before getting lighter in volume and colour towards the end of your period.

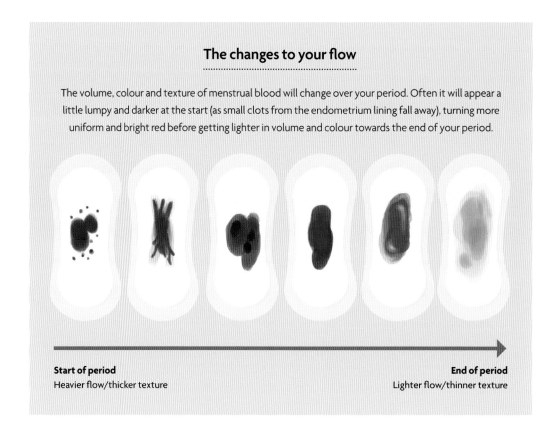

**Start of period**
Heavier flow/thicker texture

**End of period**
Lighter flow/thinner texture

## Tracking your period

From the moment you start your periods, you should begin tracking your cycle. It's a great piece of advice that I dish out to all my patients who menstruate. By keeping a record of your cycle from one month to the next, you'll get a really clear idea of your own unique pattern.

You can track your cycle by simply jotting things down in a diary or, even better, by downloading a free period tracking app onto your phone. I really can't recommend these apps enough; they're such handy little tools and are so simple to use. See the Resources section (see page 241) for more information.

Having this information to hand during a medical appointment can be extremely useful. Assessing your tracking data will help your doctor to gauge whether your cycle is imbalanced or out of sync, and will give them a much better idea of the symptoms you're experiencing and the treatment you require.

### Things to monitor

Date your period starts and stops

Blood flow (low to high)

Blood consistency (thin to thick)

Physical symptoms
(stomach cramps, headaches)

Emotional symptoms
(irritability, tearfulness)

### NOTES ON MY PERIOD

**DAY 1**

Cried at a nature programme today! Then found I'd started my period just before I went to bed.

**DAY 2**

Feeling teary on and off for much of the day. Also had stomach cramps and ache in vulva. Heavy flow with some clots.

**DAY 3**

Stomach cramps and vulva ache continued but mood much better. Flow still heavy.

**DAY 4**

Flow lighter today and cramps and vulva ache have gone. Feeling pretty tired so went to bed early.

**DAY 5**

Light flow and a couple of spots appeared on my chin.

**DAY 6**

Very light, pink spotting today.

## Period products

During their lifetime, most women will get through between 14,000 and 18,000 disposable pads, liners or tampons. There's a huge range of period products on the market these days, and deciding which type or brand best suits you can seem very daunting when you first start your periods. It's often a case of trial and error, as well as personal preference – some people choose reusable products, some choose single-use products; some people choose pads, some choose tampons, and others use a combination of both – but it should be based on what you like, what you feel comfortable with, and what you can afford or have access to.

Always read the instructions on your period products, so you know you're using them correctly, and bear in mind that leaks can occasionally occur with any type of period product. Make a habit of changing your period product regularly – every four hours or so (or each time you pass urine) is a good rule of thumb for tampons and pads. Period cups can usually last a little longer, but ensure you give them a proper clean in the sink under clean running water when you empty it and reinsert.

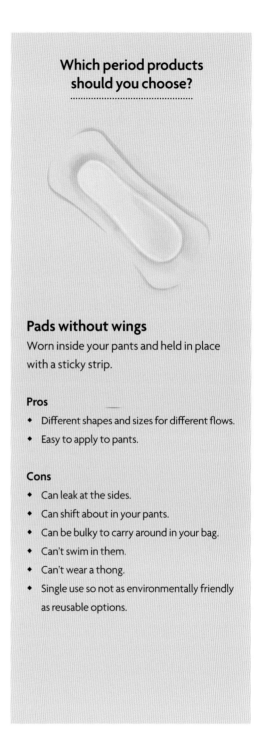

## Which period products should you choose?

## Pads without wings

Worn inside your pants and held in place with a sticky strip.

### Pros

- Different shapes and sizes for different flows.
- Easy to apply to pants.

### Cons

- Can leak at the sides.
- Can shift about in your pants.
- Can be bulky to carry around in your bag.
- Can't swim in them.
- Can't wear a thong.
- Single use so not as environmentally friendly as reusable options.

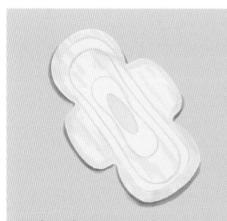

## Pads with wings

Worn inside your pants and held in place with a sticky strip and side flaps.

### Pros

- Different shapes and sizes for different flows.
- More secure in your pants than pads without wings.
- Less chance of leaking compared to pads without wings.

### Cons

- Can leak if wrong absorbency is chosen.
- Wings can cause chafing in the groin and thighs as they rub.
- Can be bulky to carry around in your bag.
- Can't swim in them.
- Can't wear a thong.
- Single use so not as environmentally friendly as reusable options.

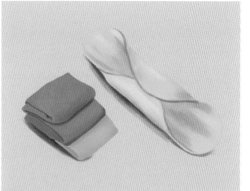

## Reusable pads

Worn inside your pants and held in place with popper fastenings.

### Pros

- Reusable, so more environmentally friendly and cost-effective in the long term.
- Different shapes and sizes for different flows.
- Easy to apply to pants.

### Cons

- Bulky to carry around in your bag.
- Will need to carry a waterproof bag for used pads if you are on the go.
- Can't swim in them.
- Can't wear a thong.

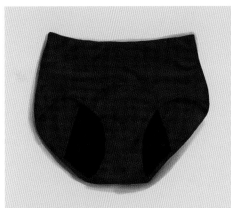

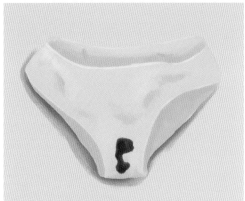

## Period pants

Underwear with additional absorbency in the gusset to keep you dry.

### Pros

- Reusable, so more environmentally friendly and cost-effective in the long term.
- Different sizes and styles for different flows.
- Can also be used alongside internal protection (period cup or tampon) for extra peace of mind on heavier days.
- Sometimes also available as a swimwear version, so you can wear during swimming.

### Cons

- More costly than regular underwear.
- Can be bulky to carry around in your bag if your flow is heavy and you are out for the whole day; carry a waterproof bag and a spare in case you need to change.

## Free bleeding

Not wearing period 'protection' and allowing menstrual blood to flow freely.

### Pros

- Can bleed as nature intended.
- No products, so environmentally friendly.
- Has been practiced for millennia and more recently used as a protest about taxes on period products, disposable period products and silencing of women's issues.

### Cons

- No protection, so can cause stains on clothing, seating and bedlinen.
- Can increase your laundry load.

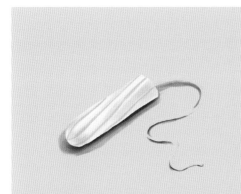

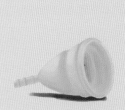

## Tampons

A soft tube that is inserted into the vagina with an applicator or finger.

**Pros**

- Different absorbencies to suit flow.
- Discreet; can fit in the palm, purse or pocket.
- Can be worn while swimming.
- The external string isn't visible once inserted.
- Can't feel the tampon once it's inside.
- Can wear with a thong.

**Cons**

- Can leak if wrong absorbency is chosen.
- Very rarely can cause toxic shock syndrome (TSS), easily prevented if changed regularly.
- Inserting a tampon can sometimes be uncomfortable (especially the first time).
- If incorrectly inserted, it can be expelled from the vaginal canal.
- Single use so not as environmentally friendly as reusable options.

## Period cup

A soft cup that is folded and inserted into the vagina to collect blood.

**Pros**

- Reusable, so more environmentally friendly and cost-effective in the long term.
- Can be left in for up to eight hours before taking out and rinsing.
- Some versions can be worn during sex.
- Can be worn while swimming.
- Can't feel the cup once it's inside.
- Can wear with a thong.

**Cons**

- Insertion can be tricky; it needs practice.
- Can be messy; you have to use your finger to fish it out before rinsing.
- Needs a thorough wash after use.
- If you have heavy flow the cup can overflow.
- If you have fibroids the cup can get in the way and be uncomfortable.

### Period products for trans & non-binary people

Much more work needs to be done by manufacturers to make period products more inclusive for trans and non-binary people who menstruate. Most pads, pants and tampons are sold in feminine-looking packaging (so lots of pink flowers, birds and butterflies) that, according to patients I speak with, can trigger their dysphoria and make them feel uncomfortable when purchasing them in shops. Because of this, many trans and non-binary people resort to buying their products online, often opting for period pants with plain designs, or period cups with gender-neutral packaging.

### Period products & the environment

Did you know that we all have our own period mountains? I used to think that liners, pads and tampon applicators were incinerated, but this isn't always the case; most of them are left sitting on our beautiful planet. I was horrified to hear from a green-minded colleague that each packet of pads contains the equivalent of four plastic bags (and we all know how long that would take to decompose).

If you can, I'd really recommend that you consider trying reusable period products like pads, pants and cups. The initial outlay may prove to be more expensive than disposable products, but in the long term it works out more cost-effective because they can last for years. And, since they're more sustainable than disposable period products, they're much better for the environment.

If you do use disposable period products, please bin them sensibly. Don't wrap a used pad in a plastic bag or reams of toilet paper because you're worried someone will see it; just roll it up and pop it in the bin.

### Period products & sport

It's quite normal for women and girls to stay active or play sport when they're menstruating. Some may prefer not to do so, which is totally fine – they could have very heavy flow, or bad period pain, and might want to take it easy – but others may find that exercise makes them feel better during their period, both physically and emotionally. For reasons of comfort and practicality, most women who participate in sport prefer to use tampons (especially if they're swimming or cycling) or reusable period-proof swimwear and shorts, but pads are perfectly suitable for low-intensity forms of exercise such as walking or pilates.

A year's worth of disposable period products contributes 5.3kg of $CO_2$

# Period inequality

Period inequality is an unequal access to period products, education and menstrual care because of boundaries of economics, ethnicity or culture. It is vital that women everywhere, regardless of their race or class, are able to access the period products and knowledge they need to experience their period each month without it inflicting on their work, education or home life.

A survey conducted in 2019 by Plan International highlighted that one in ten girls in the UK could not afford period products. During the Coronavirus pandemic this figure went up to one in three.

Some people use the expression 'period poverty' to describe the struggle faced by women who cannot access safe and affordable products. I find this terminology incredibly demeaning, and prefer not to use it. Firstly, if you can't afford food or you belong to a low-income household, the last thing you want to be labelled as is suffering from 'period poverty'. Secondly, it suggests that women are weak, powerless victims of their periods, and that this perfectly natural process is a hardship or a hindrance. Thirdly, it also belittles the deep inequality and discrimination they face in these circumstances, which often stems from race, class, gender and socio-economic status.

This pejorative terminology also implies that this problem is largely confined to developing countries, which simply isn't true. Period product inequality is a global issue – UK food banks frequently appeal for donations of pads and tampons for low-income women – and it has serious repercussions. Limited access to period products can deter girls from attending school, or women from attending work, thus restricting their educational and professional development, and earning power and opportunity. Using alternative 'protection' (like rags or toilet tissue) can lead to harmful infection and the associated blood leakages can cause shame and embarrassment.

I find it all so saddening and infuriating. Governments around the world need to get a better grip on the situation, and work more closely with women's health organizations, if we're going to put an end to this unfairness. With that in mind, my good friend Manjit Gill MBE founded Binti International, an organization that seeks to provide menstrual dignity to girls around the world (their mantra is 'availability, affordability and awareness'). She talks of the necessity of a 'period revolution' to normalize menstruation and to eradicate stigma and suffering, and has led a campaign for all business and public spaces to have free period products.

If you're having problems accessing period products, please don't suffer in silence. Speak to a health professional who may be able to signpost you to an organization that can help, or see Resources from page 241.

# Let's talk about periods

Periods are a natural and completely normal element of puberty and beyond and as a society we need to be more open about discussions around them – not just between women, but between men, women, trans and non-binary people.

While this book aims to help women and girls understand their periods, I can't emphasise enough that it's so important for *everyone* close to them, including single dads or those in same-sex relationships, to feel comfortable talking about periods with their daughters, and that they can deal with the subject openly, honestly and without embarrassment.

The good news is that attitudes among fathers could well be changing. A YouGov survey commissioned by the charity Action Aid in 2017, to mark Menstrual Hygiene Day, revealed that while nearly half (47 per cent) of daughters said they'd feel uncomfortable discussing periods with their fathers, only 9 per cent of men would feel uncomfortable discussing periods with their daughters. Half of men surveyed (50 per cent) said they wouldn't feel uncomfortable buying period protection for women, yet only 16 per cent of women said they'd feel comfortable asking a man to buy period products for them. So if we're going to continue breaking down the stigma barrier, inter-generational communication is key. Daughters, talk to your dads...and dads, talk to your daughters!

As far as I'm concerned, no age is off-limits when it comes to talking about menstruation. I think parents and carers should start discussing period-related matters with their children as early as possible, at a stage in their lives when they're able to absorb and understand reliable and sensible information. There's no hard and fast rule, of course – all children are different – but as a parent or carer, you'll know instinctively when the time is right to prompt that conversation. Try not to delay this too much. In many instances, the big 'period talk' when a child reaches high school age can often come much too late in the day. And please don't ignore the subject of menstruation completely, or rely on your child's teachers or classmates to tell them about it; I think we owe it to our daughters to open up that channel of communication within the family unit.

**The average woman in the UK will spend up to £18,450 on products geared toward her period**

Don't forget that most boys will live alongside women who menstruate – their mum, their sisters and cousins, their aunts, their grandmothers – yet, all too often, periods are never discussed openly, often as a result of shame and stigma. It doesn't have to be this way, though. The males in the household cannot fail to benefit from factual, reliable information, in order that they may better understand this perfectly normal and natural bodily function.

When your daughter starts her periods – the average age is 12, so plan to introduce the subject at an even earlier age so she isn't surprised or confused when the time comes – it's vital that she receives support from her parents and carers. This emotional and physical milestone can be a difficult, confusing and scary time, and they will really appreciate your love and understanding. Congratulate your child on this new phase of life. Prompt a conversation by asking them how they're feeling, both physically and emotionally; whether they're getting any breast tenderness or abdominal cramps, for example, or suffering with tiredness or mood swings. Just asking your daughter about their periods is beneficial in itself; ignoring it, or just brushing it off as a 'woman's problem' is not helpful and can be quite isolating for young girls who are coming to terms with their changing bodies, and who are adapting to this new phase in their lives.

There are lots of practical things you can do to help, too, not least ensuring that you have a good supply of period products for your daughter to use, or even going to the pharmacy together to buy her preferred pads or tampons. If she experiences stomach cramps, stock up the freezer with ice packs or offer to fill up a hot water bottle.

**A 2017 survey revealed that nearly half of daughters in the UK said they'd feel uncomfortable discussing periods with their fathers**

If she suffers with headaches, ensure you have enough paracetamol in the bathroom cabinet. This advice applies to boyfriends, partners and husbands as well as fathers, of course. Your other halves will thank you for it!

There's plenty more you can do to help your loved one during their menstrual cycle. Try to show understanding if they're displaying tell-tale PMS signs such as tiredness, anxiety or irritability. Deal sympathetically with any instances of period blood leaking onto clothes or bedlinen, which can be quite traumatic and upsetting (and certainly seek advice from a doctor if this happens regularly). Keep school staff, or extra-curricular club leaders, informed if your daughter is suffering with period cramps, heavy flow or severe fatigue. By acting with care and compassion, you'll help to minimize those awful feelings of shame and stigma.

# It's time to talk about periods... without shame or embarrassment!

# Cultural attitudes towards menstruation

For centuries periods have been surrounded by myths and rumours that stigmatize those who menstruate. Although improved access to education in today's society has exposed the untruth of many of these, many still prevail.

The onset of menstruation can have a huge emotional and psychological impact on a girl and a first period is seen as a significant milestone that can be associated with a 'coming of age' or 'entry into womanhood', both of which are observed communally in a Bat Mitzvah (a Jewish ritual) or a Quinceañera (a celebration in Hispanic countries that literally means 'one who is 15').

However, some communities can perceive periods as 'unclean' and as a consequence, opt to impose restrictive measures on females. In Islam, for example, women who are menstruating aren't able to pray or go to the Mosque. In Hinduism, if a woman is on her period she cannot prepare food, eat with the family or attend the temple. In some areas of rural India and Nepal, girls can be banished to customized 'period huts'. This segregation can adversely affect how a girl views her menstrual cycle, excluding her from religious events and essentially ostracizing her from her community.

In fact, a 2017 study (by the Clue period tracker app), found a remarkable number of myths and superstitions remain. In the United States many believe that using tampons may break your hymen (the thin piece of skin that partially covers your vagina) and render you 'impure' by taking away your virginal status, a ridiculous myth that is common globally. Also in the US, you (apparently) can't touch vegetables during or before the pickling process because they'll go bad. And some say you can't go camping in the wild because bears will smell the blood. Totally absurd, of course, and completely untrue!

In Israel some mothers believe that slapping their daughter in the face when she gets her first period will give her beautiful red cheeks for the rest of her life. Menstruating girls are told not to shower with hot water because it will give them a heavy flow. Needless to say, there's no evidence to support either!

In Italy, some women stay out of the kitchen during their period because their dough won't rise properly – what nonsense! – so they won't be able to produce decent bread or pizza.

In Argentina it is said that those on their period can't make whipped cream or butter because it'll curdle. Another myth tells girls not to soak in the bath because it will cause their bleeding to stop and reduce their fertility.

In India girls must wash their hair on the first day of menstruation in order to clean themselves but, for the remainder of their period, they are not allowed to wash their hair too much since their flow will reduce and their fertility will be affected. In fact, the link between hair and female health is very much a recurring theme in many faiths and cultures, including Islam and Judaism. A woman's 'crowning glory' is seen as a sign of beauty and a symbol of fertility, and many express the view that it shouldn't be excessively touched, washed or cut during their period. I beg to differ, of course.

And, to round things off, here are some other menstruation myths that I have come across: in Mexico, if you're on your period you should avoid vigorous dancing to active rhythms in order to protect your uterus; in Romania, you can't touch flowers because they'll die quicker; in Malaysia, you are told to wash your pads before throwing them out, otherwise ghosts will come back to haunt you; and in the Dominican Republic you can't paint your nails or drink lemonade. Washing your face with the blood from your first period gives you clear skin, according to a myth in the Philippines, and in Brazil, if you're menstruating you can't walk around barefoot otherwise you'll get bad cramps. In France, you're banned from making mayonnaise because it will curdle and, in Bolivia, you're told not to cradle babies because it will make them ill. None of these claims has an ounce of merit!

Some of these superstitions may sound bizarrely amusing, but there is a serious (and dangerous) side to all this myth-making. Many of them advocate behavioural restrictions that contribute to gender-biased taboos and discrimination. These entrenched falsehoods make it harder for girls to talk about their menstrual health and lead to shame and silence.

These myths and superstitions also push the idea that women, once they start their periods, are going to be ruining something, or restricted from doing something. Such misogynistic superstitions

become embedded in certain cultures and are passed on through generations, often via mothers and grandmothers, who'll perpetuate them without educating their girls about the biology of their own bodies.

People need to realize, for example, that period blood is the same blood that runs through everyone's body; it just happens to incorporate the uterus lining as well as other cell matter. Too many communities believe this blood to be 'old' or 'dirty', which is wrong and misguided; if this was the case, women would have regular infections. Period blood is clean, healthy and normal.

My friend Manjit from Bindi International also believes that much of the stigma and shame related to menstruation stems from its over-sexualization. Ideally, it should be taught in schools around the world as a stand-alone topic, and explained in such a way that empowers girls to understand themselves, and teaches boys to become empathetic and supportive.

There's also a misconception – one I've witnessed myself, with my own patients – that menstrual (and menopausal) matters are largely 'Western' issues that are only discussed and addressed among middle-class white women. This assumption may well stem from long-standing and deep-rooted socio-cultural attitudes and religious traditions. It may also stem from institutional failings within the healthcare system – and the fact that we still have so much to learn. But whatever the reason, it makes me feel sad and frustrated. Women and girls across the board should receive the same access to healthcare – regardless of creed, colour, class or culture – and, with that in mind, I've made it my long-term mission to help break down those barriers.

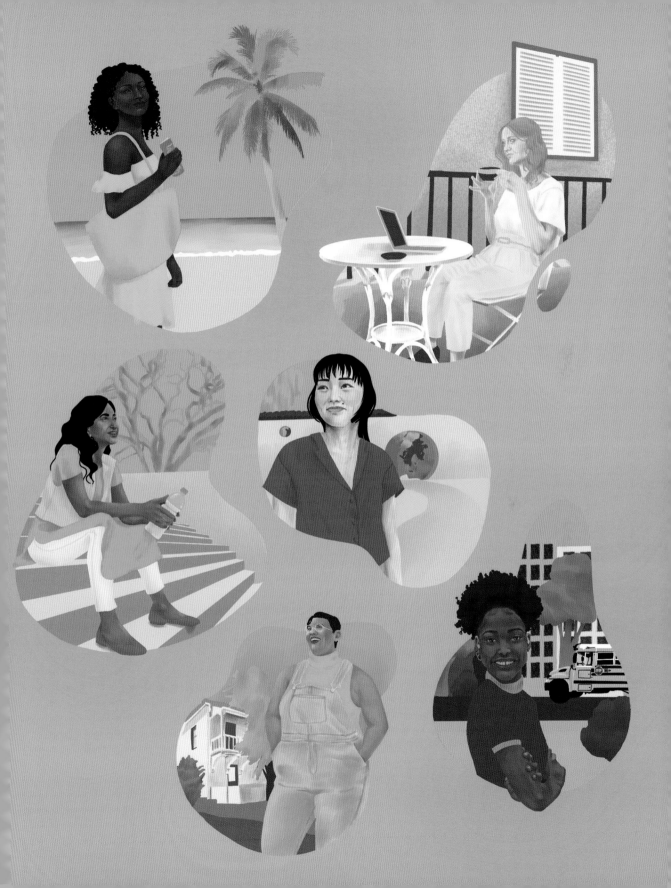

# Health & comfort issues during your monthly cycle

Some women have trouble-free menstruation cycles that impinge little on their daily lives, but many others suffer physical or emotional issues at different times in their cycle which can have a huge impact on school, work or relationships. Here are some of the common issues.

## Period pain

Period pain is no joke. It's a common but debilitating condition that should always be taken very seriously. Severe period pain is known as dysmenorrhea and some doctors are finally admitting that period cramps can be just as painful as a heart attack, if not worse, and I think they're spot on.

So why do we get period pain, and how should we deal with it? During your menstrual period, a hormone called prostaglandin – which helps the body deal with injury and illness – causes your uterus to contract in order to expel its lining. Prostaglandin is so powerful, in fact, that it triggers labour and contractions in childbirth. When the endometrial cells lining the uterus break down the during menstruation, they also release large amounts of prostaglandin. This prostaglandin constricts the blood vessels in the uterus and make the muscle layer constrict by causing contractions, which temporarily cut off blood supply to the uterus and starve it of oxygen. This causes a throbbing, cramping pain that can spread from your lower abdomen to your lower back. The effects of prostaglandin are localized, meaning they only act where they are produced, which is why most period pain is felt in the abdominal area.

Some women suffer a monthly host of intense physical symptoms that can include fever, nausea, inflammation, dizziness, clumsiness, tinnitus and even diarrhoea (otherwise known as 'period poops'). Having to deal with this multifactorial pain while coping with life, jobs and families makes women totally incredible, don't you think? The good news is that this release of prostaglandin is temporary and the body quickly starts to break it down, diminishing its effect on the body. This is the reason why, for the majority of women, period pain doesn't linger too long, usually straddling day 1 and day 3 of their cycle.

> We need to stop normalizing pain. Take paracetamol or ibuprofen to ease your symptoms, and if that doesn't work, see your doctor.

# Painful periods: What can you do to manage the pain?

Many women experience pain each month during and before their period. Don't be afraid to try the following solutions to manage it:

- **Take paracetamol** regularly (a maximum of two 500-milligram tablets, every four to six hours, no more than four times a day).

- **Take ibuprofen** (a maximum of two 200-milligram tablets, three times a day) in addition to paracetamol if necessary, and only if you are over 12 years old. Ibuprofen isn't tolerated by everyone though. It must only ever be taken with food – never on an empty stomach – so as not to trigger acid reflux, worsen asthma symptoms or interact with other medicines. There are other over-the-counter options containing ibuprofen lysine that are sold specifically to treat period pain, but they can be quite expensive, and you may find that generic ibuprofen does just as good a job.

- **Hot water bottles** can help to relieve cramps.

- **Drink plenty of fluids** to keep you hydrated.

- **Vitamin B$_1$ (thiamine)** (100 milligrams daily throughout the month) can help some people.

- **Magnesium glycinate** (300–400 milligrams at bedtime, increasing to 600 milligrams for one week before a period is due) can also be beneficial.

- **Yoga** can help you to relax and relieve cramping.

- **Acupuncture** can be of great benefit to some people.

- **Quitting smoking** is good for your health anyway, but has been found to have a positive impact on period pain.

- **Cutting down on alcohol** during your period can also have a positive impact.

- **Transcutaneous electrical nerve stimulation** machines (also known as TENS) have been flagged in some data studies as having a positive effect in helping to control and regulate pain. These are available in pharmacies or online, or to hire if you would like to try before you buy.

If you find that you need to use medical pain relief during every period, and it improves your symptoms, there's nothing to be concerned about. However, if you're unable to control your period pain despite using paracetamol and/or ibuprofen, do not hesitate to see a doctor. They will assess you to pinpoint any underlying causes and will do all they can to help ease your discomfort and improve your quality of life. Do not suffer in silence. Do not 'keep calm and carry on', despite what others might tell you. Pain can be controlled, and does not have to be endured.

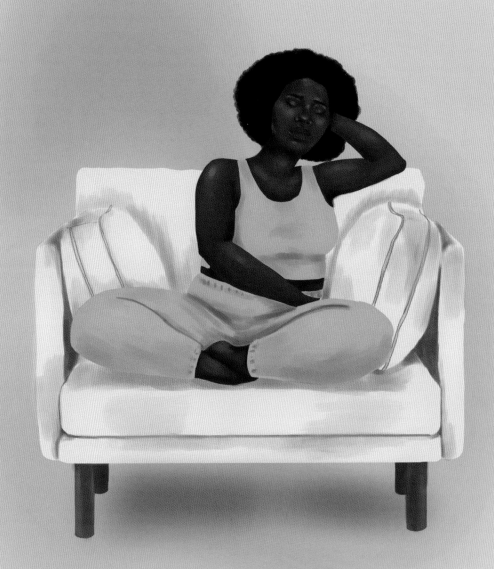

## Premenstrual syndrome

So what is PMS, and what are its effects? During your period, hormone levels can go up and down. These hormones help your body to prepare for possible pregnancy and send signals back and forth between the brain and the ovaries, causing changes to the follicles and the uterus. These hormones, as they fluctuate, are also responsible for troublesome premenstrual syndrome symptoms which can include:

- Headaches and/or migraine
- Tender and/or swollen breasts
- Abdominal bloating, pain and/or cramps
- Diarrhoea and/or constipation
- Sugar cravings
- Swollen legs
- Backache
- Fluid retention
- Fatigue, lethargy and/or excessive sleepiness
- Clumsiness
- Insomnia
- Reduced libido
- Acne
- Lowered ability to cope
- Anxiety and/or nervous tension
- Anger, aggression and/or irritability
- Impairment of concentration
- Loss of confidence
- Mood swings and/or tearfulness
- Depression

Diagnostically, PMS only requires one or two symptoms to qualify and is reported to be experienced by up to 50 per cent of women around the globe. Premenstrual tension (PMT) is essentially the same condition – you'll probably hear both PMS and PMT being referred to – although most clinicians prefer to use 'syndrome' rather than 'tension' as it's a looser, more all-encompassing definition (and, some would argue, sounds a little less emotionally charged).

In terms of treatment for PMS, your doctor will be able to suggest ways you can best manage your symptoms. Emotional and psychological issues can be eased with anti-depressants – selective serotonin reuptake inhibitors (SSRI). Being prescribed with this type of medication does not necessarily mean you're suffering with depression as they're common remedies for hormonal imbalances. Long-acting contraceptives (LARCS) such as implants (see page 77) and injections (see page 78) can also help to regulate your hormones.

Making changes to your routine and lifestyle can also be beneficial. I often encourage patients suffering with PMS to engage in exercise – an online yoga session, perhaps, or a walk in a park or the countryside – and, if they can, to cut out cigarettes and alcohol. Dietary supplements like vitamin $B_6$, vitamin D, calcium and magnesium can help to improve mood and wellbeing in some cases, as can complementary therapies (I know many patients who are devotees of acupuncture, aromatherapy and reflexology, for example). Evidence with regard to alternative therapy is scant, I admit, but if something is helping someone to cope with their PMS, and is causing no harm, I'm happy for them to continue.

For women and girls who experience PMS, the impact on schooling, work and relationships can be significant. I've treated women whose PMS has led to exam failure, career disruption, financial losses and marriage breakdown. Yet, despite the debilitating nature of this condition, society often treats it with scorn and ridicule. Comments like,

'Is it the time of the month, love?' are woven into the fabric of our culture and it needs to stop. Sufferers need to be treated with compassion, not contempt.

## Premenstrual dysphoric disorder

Premenstrual dysphoric disorder (PMDD) is a reaction in the brain to the rise and fall of oestrogen and progesterone. Symptoms can be severe and worsen over time, and can be especially prevalent around menstruation and perimenopause. PMDD symptoms can also be felt around times of pregnancy, birth and miscarriage, despite the absence of menstrual bleeds. It is a worse extension of PMS, and sometimes can be disabling.

The International Association for Premenstrual Disorders (IAPMD) states that a diagnosis of PMDD must include one of the four core symptoms:

- Emotional changes, such as extreme mood swings, tearfulness, sudden extreme sadness or increased sensitivity to rejection, which can disrupt daily life and damage relationships
- Irritability and/or anger, perhaps including increased conflict with family and friends
- Depressed mood, or suicidal thoughts
- Feeling hopeless or worthless
- Anxiety and tension, or feelings of being on edge or 'keyed up'

A PMDD diagnosis should also include the presence of at least five of these symptoms:

- Difficulty concentrating, focusing, or thinking; brain fog
- Decreased interest in usual activities (work, school, friends, hobbies)
- Tiredness or low energy

- Changes in appetite, food cravings or over-eating
- Bloating or weight gain
- Insomnia
- Feeling out of control
- Breast tenderness
- Joint or muscle pain

PMDD is diagnosed by tracking symptoms and these should be recorded daily for at least two menstrual cycles (again, yet another good reason to track your periods – see page 47). There is also a 'self-screen' test available on the IAMPD website (see Resources from page 241) that allows you to input your symptoms. Bringing the resulting data to your healthcare appointment would be extremely helpful.

PMDD can be treated with SSRI anti-depressants, the combined oral contraceptive pill, or gonadotropin releasing hormone analogues (GnRHa) that involve monthly injections to manage the condition. Ovulation suppressants such as transdermal oestrogen or cyclical progesterone can help, as can cognitive behavioural therapy (CBT). In some circumstances an abdominal hysterectomy (the removal of the uterus) will be necessary.

I fear there's a lack of understanding regarding PMDD among some healthcare professionals, and there's no doubt that more medical research is needed. The IAMPD website contains an extensive treatment plan that people and clinicians can familiarize themselves with and, on a larger scale, I'm hoping that more detailed studies will be commissioned to discover more about this debilitating condition.

## Food cravings

So why do we have food cravings just before or during our periods? During the luteal phase (when our ovaries have released an egg, before our period starts) we experience a fluctuation in hormones, which often includes a dip in serotonin levels. Sometimes referred to as the 'happy hormone', serotonin is a chemical that can help to control appetite, sleep, sexual desire, body temperature and social behaviour. Eating carbohydrates (so that's broadly sugary, starchy and fibre-based foods) serves to boost these serotonin levels, hence why those PMS sufferers who feel tired and tetchy will find themselves reaching out for bread, biscuits and chocolate bars!

I don't have a massive problem with people satisfying their carb cravings, within reason (as a cake-lover myself, the occasional slice of Victoria sponge never fails to cheer me up if I'm feeling low!). However, to counter balance the odd lapse – and to help keep your cravings under control – try to choose a varied and balanced diet that's rich in fruit, vegetables, whole grains and calcium.

## Heavy periods

While many people who menstruate won't have severe period-related problems, others aren't so lucky. Heavy periods (medically known as menorrhagia) can massively impact your quality of life, and should not have to be endured. Fear of leakages can deter many women from attending school or work, and prevent them participating in the things they enjoy, like sport or socializing.

I always treat this condition with the utmost seriousness. I often refer patients for an ultrasound scan, which may ascertain why they're bleeding so heavily, and can check for conditions like fibroids, endometriosis, adenomyosis and polycystic ovary syndrome (all of these issues are covered in Phase 2 of this book, starting on page 96). Once the cause has been pinpointed we can help manage the bleeding with tablets such as tranexamic acid or mefenamic acid (the latter tends to be prescribed if you have associated pain, too).

Then, if my patient isn't planning to get pregnant, I can prescribe the combined oral contraceptive pill or the progesterone-only mini-pill (see page 76). If that's not suitable, other options include a contraceptive implant or injection (see pages 77 and 78) or the progesterone IUS coil (see page 79). If you've never had a baby, the Jaydess™ or Kyleena™ progesterone-only coil (or 'mini coil') may be prescribed. In extremely severe cases, a patient may be referred to a specialist gynaecologist to discuss the possibility of a hysterectomy (removal of the uterus).

If you are using a new pad or tampon hourly or more, then don't suffer in silence. We shouldn't normalize heavy bleeding and your doctor may be able to help.

### Anaemia & periods

Anaemia is a condition characterized by low levels of haemoglobin (iron) in the red blood cells that make up blood. Red blood cells carry oxygen around your body from your lungs, so they're vital for all bodily functions. Your bone marrow constantly needs iron to make new blood cells to replace older ones that have become worn out or have been lost due to bleeding. However, with frequent bleeding, your body runs low on iron and can't quite keep up in making enough new red blood cells to maintain normal functions. This can lead to the following symptoms:

- Shortness of breath (especially when exercising)
- Palpitations (heart racing)
- Feeling faint
- Looking pale
- Tiredness

A low intake of iron can contribute to anaemia; this can stem from a vegan or vegetarian diet, for example, or from undiagnosed coeliac disease (poor iron absorption is a feature of the latter). Anaemia can also be caused by periods – especially if they're heavy – and affects approximately ten per cent of menstruating women. So, if you have symptoms that are suggestive of anaemia, please make an appointment to see your doctor. They'll assess you fully before performing a simple blood test to measure your blood count and check for coeliac disease. If you are indeed diagnosed with anaemia, this can be corrected by prescribed iron tablets to allow your body to produce enough red blood cells. If you have heavy periods but have not been diagnosed with anaemia, then an over-the-counter supplement of 17–20 milligrams a day could help.

*Always seek help if you're worried about your menstrual health.*

### Other period-related issues

It's worth talking to a doctor if any of the issues opposite apply to you. Again – and I can't stress this enough – please consider keeping a diary or downloading a tracker app as this will really improve the quality of the consultation with a healthcare professional.

**29%**
of women of reproductive age are affected by anaemia

# Puberty & periods: What symptoms might warrant a visit to your doctor?

Puberty and periods are a natural part of growing up, but be aware that sometimes you will need more medical advice. In particular, if you:

- **Have started a period** and you're aged between seven and nine.
- **Have not yet had a period** and you're aged 16 or above.
- **Haven't yet had a period but developed breasts** more than three years ago.
- **Haven't had any further periods for two years** since your first period.
- **Are not menstruating regularly** every three to six weeks.
- **Have missed three periods in a row**, or gone 90 days without a period.
- **Have extremely heavy bleeding** – sometimes called flooding – that soaks through a pad or a tampon (especially if it has to be changed more frequently than every four hours).
- **Frequently pass large blood clots** (larger than 2.5cm).
- **Have periods that last between seven and ten days**, as a regular occurrence.
- **Have severe PMS/PMDD** symptoms (see pages 63 and 64).
- **Have severe cramps** that aren't improved by taking simple pain relief, such as paracetamol or ibuprofen.

All women, regardless of age, should also seek medical advice if they experience any vaginal bleeding that seems out of the ordinary, such as:

- **Between periods**
- **After sex**
- **After the menopause** (if bleeding restarts after one year of no periods)
- **Heavier and more painful** than usual, especially if you also have symptoms of anaemia (tiredness, looking pale, feeling faint, palpitations/heart racing, shortness of breath – particularly during exercise).

Abnormal bleeding can be a key symptom of three gynaecological cancers (uterus, cervical and vaginal – see page 150) and is a less common symptom of ovarian cancer. It may also be an indicator of other conditions like endometriosis, adenomyosis, polycystic ovary syndrome (PCOS) and fibroids. In girls and younger women, it's commonly understood that the risk of cancer is lower – but if you have any concerns at all, don't hesitate to seek medical advice.

# Violence against women & girls

The United Nations defines violence against women and girls (VAWG) as 'gender-based violence that results in, or is likely to result in, physical, sexual or psychological harm or suffering to women, including threats of such acts, coercion or arbitrary deprivation of liberty, whether occurring in public or in private life.'

It's a sad fact that most clinicians, including myself, have encountered patients across the spectrum of age and gender who have experienced abuse or violence. Doctors are trained to recognize the signs (the person may well see the surgery as a 'safe space') and will treat these individuals with the utmost care and sensitivity. Referrals to specialist clinics, services and relevant authorities may occur; these 'multi-agency' approaches are often the most effective way to address the issue.

In an ideal world, human relationships would be positive and pleasurable experiences, free from any coercion, discrimination or violence. Sexual intercourse should only happen in a consensual situation, one in which you feel totally happy and comfortable. You must not feel pressured or threatened to do anything against your will, and you have every right to say no, to exit a situation and to seek a place of refuge.

If you are a victim of any physical, psychological or sexual abuse – including sex trafficking, so-called 'honour' abuse, or intimate image abuse (also known as revenge porn) – please ask for help. You can reach out to a trusted friend or family member, your doctor, a police officer, a charity helpline or website. I appreciate that stepping forward and speaking up is easier said than done, but rest assured there's a great deal of advice and support available (see Resources from page 241).

## Female genital mutilation

Female genital mutilation (FGM) is an abhorrent practice involving the ritualistic cutting of a girl's genitalia (usually her clitoris and/or labia) for 'cultural', non-medical reasons. The practice was outlawed in the UK in 1985, but FGM still takes place around the world. Globally millions of girls remain at risk, most of them of school age.

The physical, mental, sexual and emotional ramifications of FGM are manifold, and include chronic pain, repeated infections and post-traumatic stress disorder (PTSD). The practice can have chronic implications to a woman's wellbeing, and even result in death. Safeguarding patients will always be of paramount importance to doctors, so if an affected individual presents themselves to a surgery we offer them care and attention before organizing referrals to the appropriate medical and/or social services. If the patient is under 18 it is also our legal obligation to inform the police. If you, or someone else, is at risk please seek help.

FGM is child abuse, pure and simple, and it has no place in today's society. Help, advice and support is available from a number of charitable organizations (see Resources from page 241).

# Caring for your vulva & vagina

Just like the rest of your body, your genitals need lots of TLC and it's vitally important that you keep that area healthy in order to avoid fungal and bacterial infections. You should also be aware of your vaginal discharge in order to spot when something is amiss.

The following is a list of personal hygiene recommendations to help keep your vulva and vagina healthy:

- **Wash your genitals** with clear water and mild, plain soap. Your vulva does not need to smell of flowers. Soap and water are all you need, trust me.
- **Avoid perfumed soaps, gels and oils**, and don't even think about using bath bombs…they should be banned in my opinion! Many highly fragranced products use an alcohol base that can make skin dry and sensitive. This in turn disrupts candida in the vulva and can lead to yeast infections and UTIs.
- **Shower** instead of having a bath, to avoid scented bath products around the vulval area.
- **Don't use fragranced wipes** as they can upset the healthy balance of pH and bacteria inside the vagina.
- **Don't use abrasive, fragranced toilet tissue**, and rinse with clear water if you can.
- **Avoid 'douching'** (a device that pushes a stream of water into the vagina).
- **Use mild laundry detergent** to wash your underwear.
- **Avoid wearing tight clothing** and skinny jeans (the bane of my life in my surgery!) as they can trigger vulval irritation.
- **Wear cotton** underwear rather than synthetic – so avoid nylon and polyester – and try to avoid thongs.
- **Avoid wearing underwear in bed**, if possible, although this may not be practical during your period.
- **Change your period protection** regularly.
- **Use a barrier method of contraception** (such as condoms).
- **Pass urine after sex** as it flushes away any cross contamination from the perineal rectal area to the vagina and urethra and can help to prevent urinary tract infections (UTIs).
- **Avoid hot tubs**, they can be a breeding ground for bacteria and viruses.
- **Maintain a healthy weight** through nutritious diet and regular exercise.
- **Get to know the triggers** – such as sexual intercourse or your period – that can result in infections.

I know this will be a hard sell for many readers, but I would like to make a particular plea for you to avoid fragranced bath, shower and cleansing products, including those labelled 'feminine' or 'intimate'. Many contain ingredients that disturb the natural balance of vulval and vaginal bacteria and, in my opinion, do much more harm than good. For decades, beauty industry marketing and advertising campaigns have pushed the narrative that women can only keep themselves fresh by using fragranced products, the implication being that female genitals in their natural state are unclean and unhygienic. This fallacy – all too often perpetuated by misogynistic insults about smelly vaginas – is incredibly unhelpful. Wash with water and plain soap is the advice I give to all my patients with vaginas, and it's the advice I'm giving to you, too. So pass it on…

## Vaginal discharge

Vaginal discharge is a perfectly normal part of women's health – we all experience it – yet we don't pay nearly enough attention to it. It's one of those hush-hush topics that no one seems to talk about but, surprise, surprise, I have no such qualms! Monitoring your secretions means any noticeable changes can prompt you to raise concerns. The frequency and consistency of discharge can vary quite significantly, but colour and odour are clear indications of vaginal health:

* **Clear, relatively odourless discharge** is normal around pregnancy and ovulation, especially if you have had a coil inserted.

* **Whiteish discharge** is usually healthy, but if it has a lumpy consistency, and is accompanied by a burning sensation or itchiness, it might signify a yeast infection.

* **Yellowy-green discharge** is more than likely the result of an STD (see page 87).

* **Greyish discharge, with a fishy smell** is a common indicator of bacterial vaginosis (see page 71).

* **Pink-tinged discharge** suggests cervical bleeding or vaginal irritation.

* **Red and bloody discharge** signals either normal menstrual flow or, in some cases, a cervical infection or detached polyp (a type of internal growth).

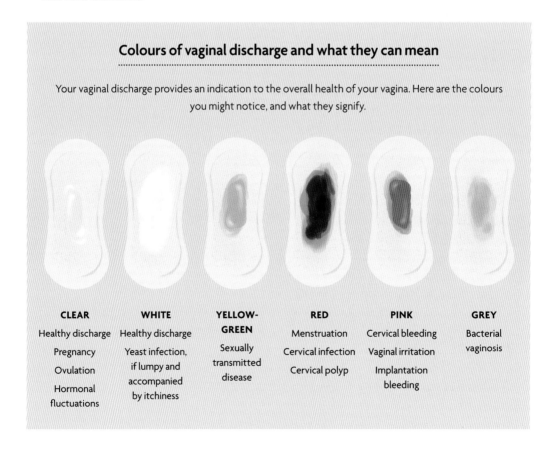

## Colours of vaginal discharge and what they can mean

Your vaginal discharge provides an indication to the overall health of your vagina. Here are the colours you might notice, and what they signify.

| **CLEAR** | **WHITE** | **YELLOW-GREEN** | **RED** | **PINK** | **GREY** |
|---|---|---|---|---|---|
| Healthy discharge | Healthy discharge | Sexually transmitted disease | Menstruation | Cervical bleeding | Bacterial vaginosis |
| Pregnancy | Yeast infection, if lumpy and accompanied by itchiness | | Cervical infection | Vaginal irritation | |
| Ovulation | | | Cervical polyp | Implantation bleeding | |
| Hormonal fluctuations | | | | | |

# Infections of the genitals & urinary tract

Like any other part of the body, the genitals can become infected and minor infections are common and usually easily treatable. Don't suffer in silence. Visit your doctor or pharmacist if you experience the symptoms of these infections. As the urinary tract is situated so close to the anus in female anatomy, infections of this area can be common.

## Genital infections

Bacterial vaginosis and thrush are the most common infections that affect the genital area.

Bacterial vaginosis is a common condition that can affect anyone with a vagina from puberty to menopause, particularly those who are sexually active (although it is not a sexually transmitted disease). It is usually caused by a change in the natural pH balance of the bacteria in the vulva and vagina, and signs to watch out for include a thin, watery white-grey vaginal discharge, which can have a fishy odour. Many women have the condition without any symptoms, but if you do have them, you may want to get hold of an over-the-counter test kit from your pharmacy. Bacterial vaginosis generally doesn't cause itching or soreness, so if you notice those symptoms I'd suggest you get checked out for thrush or a sexually transmitted disease (see page 87).

Making certain changes to your daily routine can help the symptoms (see page 69), but if things don't improve, your doctor can prescribe antibiotic tablets, gels or creams. If you have a same-sex partner, or share sex toys with someone, you both might need treating. Bacterial vaginosis can sometimes return three months after treatment and, if you are affected more than twice in a month, a longer course of antibiotics may be required.

Thrush is an infection, not a sexually transmitted disease, and is caused by an overgrowth of the *Candida albicans* yeast in the vulval and vaginal area. It's a very common condition that can occur at any age, and can be triggered by many factors, including stress, damage to the skin or poorly controlled diabetes. Thrush is more likely to affect women around ovulation, after sex, or during pregnancy; I myself have suffered with horrendous thrush during all three of my pregnancies – it made me utterly miserable – so I know exactly how awful it can feel. The classic signs are vulval/vaginal soreness and itching – which can often get worse at night – and, sometimes, a cottage cheese-like discharge.

Effective over-the-counter treatment for thrush – a cream and a pessary – can be obtained from your local pharmacy (you can buy self-tests, too). This treatment is effective, but it can take one to two weeks to work properly. If you are having unprotected sex with a male partner, it's wise for him to get treated too; men can carry the yeast, sometimes without symptoms, and can re-infect their partner during sex. He will need to apply the cream onto his penis and foreskin.

## Urinary tract infections

Urinary tract infections (UTIs) are incredibly common among girls and women because the urogenital anatomy is in close proximity to the anal area. This means that cross contamination of bugs from the back passage – *E. coli* that lives in the bowel, for example – can easily be transmitted to the bladder, kidneys or urethra (the tube through which urine leaves the body). Cystitis is the name given to inflammation of the bladder, either due to an infectious or non-infectious cause. If bacteria travel up to the kidneys, a condition called pyelonephritis may be triggered.

UTIs can be painful and distressing but the sooner you recognize the following signs and symptoms, the quicker you'll get treated:

- Burning, stinging or pain when passing urine
- Passing urine more frequently
- Passing small amounts of urine
- Passing more urine than usual during the night
- Irritation to the urethra
- Lower abdominal pain
- Lower back pain
- Raised temperature, fever and/or shivers
- Confusion and disorientation
- Nausea and/or vomiting

My advice is to keep a track of your symptoms, drink plenty of water, take paracetamol (a maximum of two 500-milligram tablets, every four to six hours, no more than four times a day) or ibuprofen if tolerated (two 200-milligram tablets, three times a day with food), and use a cold pack on your abdomen to help with the pain. For cystitis, you can buy an over-the-counter treatment in the form of sachets of crystals that are diluted in water; some people find that drinking cranberry juice relieves their symptoms, too.

If you feel you need medical intervention, contact your healthcare provider; if you're given an appointment you'll probably be asked to collect a urine sample, which will be sent to a laboratory to check for bacteria. Your doctor may then prescribe antibiotics to treat the UTI as quickly as possible, although we prefer to be in possession of your results before we do so.

### How to prevent UTIs

Recurrent UTIs are common, but the following considerations may help prevent them:

- **Always wipe yourself from front to back** (from vagina to anus) after you've been to the toilet.
- **Only use plain soap and clear water** to wash your genitals, and avoid fragranced products.
- **Consider avoiding jacuzzis**, hot tubs and baths, as they can increase the risk of UTIs.
- **Pass urine immediately after sexual intercourse** to clear out your urinary tract.
- **Take D-mannose** (a sugar available to buy as a powder or a tablet) every day. It is widely available in health food shops.
- **Drink cranberry juice** every day.
- **Consume probiotics** (lactobacillus), such as sauerkraut, kefir or probiotic yoghurts every day. These contain good bacteria that help the immune system, support gut health and help the body fight off infections, including UTIs.
- **Take topical vaginal oestrogen** if you are perimenopausal or postmenopausal, and are getting recurrent UTIs due to vaginal atrophy (see page 168).
- **Prescribed prophylactic (preventative) antibiotics** from your doctor can stop the infections.

# Sexual health & contraception

Firstly, remember that sexual health and contraception are two different elements to consider when you are sexually active. Although there is a lot of crossover between the two, contraception is to prevent pregnancy, while good sexual health practices should reduce your chances of contracting a sexually transmitted infection.

Maintaining good sexual health, and practising safe sex, is a fundamental part of a person's wellbeing. It's a perfectly natural element of everyday life that needs to be discussed honestly and openly without any shame or embarrassment. Previous generations may well have skirted around the subject – talking in riddles about the birds and the bees and the stork that delivers babies – but time has moved on, thank goodness. Nowadays everyone should have the confidence to speak freely and frankly about penises, vaginas, intercourse and condoms.

By having an honest conversation about sex and contraception – with your doctor, school nurse, sexual health practitioner, or relatives you feel comfortable with – you're being extremely sensible and responsible to yourself and any partners that you may have. If you're forearmed and forewarned you'll be less likely to contract (and pass on) harmful sexually transmitted diseases (STDs), and will be more aware of reproductive issues and contraception options (or 'family planning' as it's commonly known).

If you're thinking about engaging in sexual activity for the first time, please be sure in your mind that you feel emotionally and physically ready. If that's the case – and you're not planning to get pregnant – you'll need to research the contraception options available to you. This important fact-finding mission can take the form of a discussion with your doctor or a sexual health nurse, preferably with your partner in tow (it takes two to tango, as they say!). You can also obtain useful information from other trustworthy sources. I always advise my patients to come to their appointment armed with notes and research, since it helps them to make an informed choice, and helps me to tailor their options. It also allows them to make the most of their ten-minute slot, which can pass by very quickly. Reading the next few pages of this book may be helpful to you, I hope, but there is a wealth of information available online (see Resources from page 241).

> Be aware that human papillomavirus can be contracted through oral sex so you should use a dental dam contraception if you are practicing oral sex on a vulva with a new partner.

If you're under the age of 16 you are able to visit the doctor alone – this applies to any medical appointment, if that's what you prefer – but in these circumstances your doctor will carefully consider whether you, as a minor, have the ability to make your own independent decisions without parental consent or involvement. The healthcare professional will apply what's called the Gillick competence and Fraser guidelines (see Resources from page 241) to decide this.

A good doctor will adopt a sensitive and non-judgemental approach when discussing contraception and sexual health with all their patients, whatever their age, gender, sexuality or background. Everybody's needs and preferences will differ – individuals belonging to certain faiths and cultures may hold particular views on contraception and family planning, for example – and that should always be respected.

# 27%
## of couples practicing the withdrawal method will get pregnant each year

## Hormonal contraception

If you choose a hormonal method of contraception (either the combined pill, progesterone-only pill, contraceptive injection or implant, or the IUS coil) then it's important to consider that there may be some side effects in the initial stages as your body adjusts. In the vast majority of cases any side effects are minor. Some, such as lighter periods, reduced acne, reduced PMS, may be positive. However, you should keep track of any new symptoms you experience.

These may include:
- Fatigue
- Nausea
- Indigestion
- Constipation
- Difficulty passing urine
- Pain during sexual intercourse
- Bleeding after sexual intercourse
- Weight gain
- Mood changes.

Don't hesitate to see your doctor if you need further advice and reassurance.

## A note on the withdrawal method & emergency contraception

I will also discuss some methods – the withdrawal method and emergency contraception – that aren't long-term contraceptives but that can lessen chances of pregnancy (see the yellow panels on pages 85 and 86), which I know many couples do practice. However, you need to be clear about the failure rates of these types of practices to prevent pregnancy, which are much higher than those when preventative contraception is used.

# Which contraceptive products should you choose?

Contraceptives include hormonal options (that prevent your body preparing for pregnancy), barrier methods (that prevent sperm from reaching your vagina), or longer-term medical procedures. On the following pages I have described all the main options and how they work.

## The combined contraceptive pill

✓ Can reduce heavy periods and cramps
✓ Over 99% effective in preventing pregnancy if taken correctly
✗ Does not provide protection against STDs

There are many brands, but all contain two hormones – oestrogen and progesterone – and work by stopping the ovaries releasing an egg each month. The usual routine sees women taking one tablet each day for three weeks, and then not taking any for one week of each cycle. The packaging comes labelled with the days of the week for ease of use. In some cases, this regime can be adjusted by your doctor or sexual health nurse to help with period control, period pain and period flow. You may be able to take the Pill continuously for three months, for example, then have a four-day break.

### Pros

The combined oral pill is very effective at preventing pregnancy. It regulates menstrual cycles – it often makes them lighter – and can also decrease period cramps. For those who experience heavy menstrual flow, the Pill can help to prevent iron deficiency anaemia (low red blood cell levels). It's also thought to reduce the likelihood of ovarian and uterine cancer, ovarian cysts and pelvic inflammatory disease (PID, see page 144). Certain types can also be used as a treatment for acne.

### Cons

You need to take a tablet at the same time every day (I advise patients to put a reminder on their phone), and its effectiveness can be reduced if you suffer with prolonged vomiting and/or diarrhoea. It can't be used by everyone – it may not be prescribed to women who are obese or who smoke heavily, for example – and possible side effects can include nausea, headaches, strokes and blood clots. The pill can also affect your libido, your mood and cause weight gain. It doesn't protect against STDs, either, so you'll still need to use a condom if you have multiple partners or a new partner.

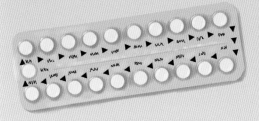

## The progesterone-only pill

✓ Can reduce heavy periods and cramps
✓ Over 99% effective in preventing pregnancy if taken correctly
✗ Must be taken at the same time each day
✗ Does not provide protection against STDs

The progesterone-only pill (POP), also known as the mini-pill, is available over the counter under various brand names. The POP contains only one hormone, progesterone, and works by thickening the cervical mucus and preventing the sperm reaching the egg. The packaging comes labelled with the days of the week for ease of use.

There's a strict time window in which the POP must be taken each day if you are having unprotected sex. There are essentially two groups of POP:
Group 1 must be taken within 12 hours of the same time each day.
Group 2, the traditional POP, must be taken within three hours of the same time each day.

### Pros

The POP shares similar advantages with the combined contraceptive pill (see page 75) but, since it only has one hormone, it offers less of a risk regarding clots and migraines. Some mini-pills may help with period cramps and PMS (your doctor will tell you more) and it is also safe to take while breastfeeding. Some brands (containing norethindrone acetate or dienogest) are used to treat endometriosis symptoms (see page 136). If taken correctly, it is more than 99 per cent effective.

### Cons

You need to take a tablet at the same time every day (I advise patients to put a reminder on their phone), and its effectiveness can be reduced if you suffer with prolonged vomiting and/or diarrhoea. Side effects from this medication may include acne, nausea, lower libido, mood swings, breast tenderness/swelling and increased vaginal discharge. In some patients with hypermobility, progesterone-only contraception can make their symptoms, such as joint pain, worse. As with the combined pill, it will not protect you against STDs so you'll need to use a condom if you have multiple partners or a new partner.

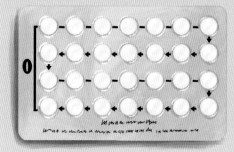

## The contraceptive implant

✓ Over 99% effective in preventing pregnancy

✓ Can cause fewer or lighter periods

✓ Once inserted, it lasts for three years so you don't need to remember to take a tablet

✓ A good option for women who can't use oestrogen-based contraception

✗ Does not provide protection against STDs

The implant is a small, bendy plastic rod that a doctor or nurse inserts beneath the skin of your upper arm. It lasts for three years, and stops you from getting pregnant by releasing progesterone into the bloodstream.

**Pros**

The implant is over 99 per cent effective, so it protects you very well against pregnancy. As it's a long-term contraceptive, you won't have to think about it for another three years (and you won't have to worry about forgetting a pill). It's a good option for women who can't use contraception that contains oestrogen, and it may also cause fewer or lighter menstrual periods.

**Cons**

Insertion involves minor surgery, which is off-putting to some, and there's a small risk of infection following the procedure. The implant may give you side effects that can include acne, depression, hair loss, weight gain and disrupted menstrual periods. It doesn't protect against STDs, either, so you'll still need to use a condom if you have multiple partners or a new partner.

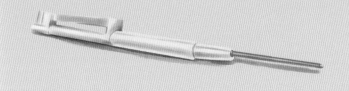

## Contraceptive injection

✓ 99% effective in preventing pregnancy
✓ Lasts for three months so you don't need to remember to take a tablet
✓ A good option for women who can't use oestrogen-based contraception
✗ Does not provide protection against STDs

The contraceptive injection is administered by a healthcare professional. Each injection contains a dose of progesterone and provides three months of protection against pregnancy. It works by thinning the lining of the endometrium and increasing the thickness of the cervical mucus, therefore not allowing sperm to reach the egg, so avoiding fertilization and implantation.

### Pros
The injection is an excellent contraceptive method (it's 99 per cent effective) and is suitable for those who can't be given oestrogen, as well as those who might worry about forgetting to take a tablet every day. Some women may stop getting menstrual periods, which may come as a relief, and studies have shown that it can help to protect against uterine cancer. As with the Pill and the coil, it doesn't interrupt sexual activity.

### Cons
Reported side effects have included tiredness and weight gain. Some studies have shown that continuous use of the contraceptive injection for more than two years can lead to bone density loss, therefore an annual review and assessment by your doctor is necessary; they may recommend an alternative method of contraception if you have risk factors such as having anorexia nervosa (an eating disorder) or being on corticosteroid therapy (for autoimmune conditions, or rheumatoid arthritis, for example).

Some women may have irregular menstrual bleeding or spotting for up to six months after the injection, occasionally for even longer. In some patients with hypermobility, progesterone-only contraception can make their symptoms, such as joint pain, worse. You need to make a note to visit the doctor every three months to get the injection topped up. It doesn't protect against STDs so you'll still need to use a condom if you have multiple partners or a new partner.

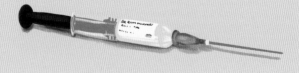

# The IUS coil

✓  Over 99% effective in preventing pregnancy
✓  Inserted by a healthcare professional so you don't have to worry about remembering it
✗  Does not provide protection against STDs

The IUS (intra-uterine system) coil is a hormone-releasing, small, T-shaped implement inserted into the uterus. It releases small amounts of progesterone into the uterus, which alters the cervical mucus and makes it difficult for sperm to survive and reach the egg. It sometimes stops ovulation and helps to reduce blood flow to the endometrium, so periods can be less heavy and painful.

**Pros**
The IUS coil is extremely effective, it only has a 0.2 per cent failure rate each year. A mini progesterone coil is also available that might be more comfortable for some people. Once inserted, the IUS can be kept in for five years, providing long-term protection without needing daily attention or regular checks. It's comfortable – neither you nor your partner will feel it's there – and some women find it lessens (or even stops) menstrual flow and prevents worsening of endometriosis. The IUS can also prevent fluctuations in hormones, which can improve symptoms of PMS and PMDD. This particular coil may also be a good option for women who have previously suffered blood clots, pulmonary embolism (PE) or deep vein thrombosis (DVT, see page 119). The Mirena™

IUS coil can also be used as the progesterone component of hormone replacement therapy for five years (see page 202).

**Cons**
The procedure can be painful, but it only five to ten minutes, and there are a number of pain relief methods that can be used, such as taking paracetamol and ibuprofen an hour before the procedure, your doctor applying a local anaesthetic gel when inserting the speculum and applying a 10 per cent lidocaine spray to the cervix. In some cases, a cervical block (a local anaesthetic injection) can be administered.

There is a slight risk of infection in the first 20 days after insertion, and there's a small chance (0.5–0.8 per cent) of it falling out (the risk varies, but it is slightly higher in 14–19-year-olds or for patients with Ehlers-Danlos Syndrome/hypermobility). There is an even smaller risk of it puncturing the uterus. In some patients with hypermobility, progesterone-only contraception can make their symptoms worse. It doesn't protect against STDs so you'll need to use a condom if you have multiple partners or a new partner.

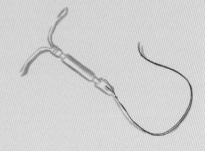

## The Vaginal Ring

✓ Over 99% effective in preventing pregnancy if used correctly
✓ Self-inserted once a month so you don't have to worry about remembering it daily
✗ Does not provide protection against STDs

The vaginal ring, sometimes referred to as a NuvaRing™, is a soft plastic ring that releases a continual dose of oestrogen and progestogen. This works in the same way as the combined contraceptive pill to prevent pregnancy by stopping the ovaries from releasing an egg each month. It is inserted into the vagina with your fingers and should then be kept in place for 21 days. After 21 days it is removed from the vagina and left out for 7 days, which will lead to a monthly bleed. After 7 days a new ring should be inserted and the cycle continues.

### Pros

If used correctly, the vaginal ring is extremely effective in preventing pregnancy, and if you insert it within 5 days of the start of your period, it will be effective straight away. It is suitable for people who are confident they will remember the routine of when to insert and remove it but don't want to remember to take a daily pill. As with other hormonal options, it can make periods lighter and less painful, and reduce PMS symptoms. If you would prefer not to have a monthly bleed then you can insert a new ring straight after removing the old one, or have a shorter break (than 7 days) between rings.

### Cons

You need to remember when to insert it and when to remove it each month. If you start using it more than 5 days after the start of your period you will also need to use additional contraception until the ring has been inserted for 7 days. It can't be used by everyone – it may not be prescribed to women who are overweight or who smoke, for example – and possible side effects can include nausea, headaches, strokes and blood clots. Some people and their partners can feel the ring during sex, this does not mean it is inserted incorrectly however. Occasionally the ring can come out on its own. If this happens you should re-insert the ring (if it happens in the first week) or insert a new ring (if it happens in week two or three) and use additional contraception for 7 days. Prescriptions are usually available as a batch of 4 months' worth so you will need fairly regular trips to your doctor or sexual health clinic to renew the prescription. It doesn't protect against STDs so you'll need to use a condom if you have multiple partners or a new partner.

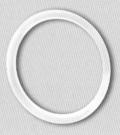

## The IUD coil

✓ Over 99% effective in preventing pregnancy
✓ Inserted by a healthcare professional so you don't have to worry about remembering it or taking it correctly
✓ A good option for women who want very reliable contraception without taking hormones
✗ Does not provide protection against STDs

The IUD (intra-uterine device) coil is a small, T-shaped implement that is inserted into the uterus. It does not contain any hormones but releases a small amount of copper into the uterus, which weakens sperm and stops it from reaching an egg.

### Pros

The IUD coil is extremely effective in preventing pregnancy, it has only a 0.1 per cent failure rate each year. Once inserted, it can remain in place for ten years so provides long-term protection and doesn't require daily attention or regular checks; you just leave it in situ. It's comfortable – neither you nor your partner will feel it's there – and is a great option for women who've had breast cancer and need to avoid hormones.

### Cons

As with the IUS coil, the procedure can be painful, but it takes only five to ten minutes, and there are a number of pain relief methods that can be used, such as taking paracetamol and ibuprofen an hour before the procedure, your doctor applying a local anaesthetic gel when inserting the speculum and applying a 10 per cent lidocaine spray to the cervix. In some cases, a cervical block (a local anaesthetic injection) can be administered, but for some women the needle can cause pain.

There is a slight risk of infection in the first 20 days after coil insertion, and there's a small chance (0.5–0.8 per cent) of it falling out (the risk varies, but studies have shown it is slightly higher in 14–19-year-olds, in patients with Ehlers-Danlos Syndrome, a connective tissue disorder, and if it's inserted immediately after a vaginal birth). There is an even smaller risk of a coil puncturing the uterus. The copper coil can have some side effects, including longer and heavier periods, increased cramping and occasional spotting. It doesn't protect against STDs so you'll need to use a condom if you have multiple partners or a new partner.

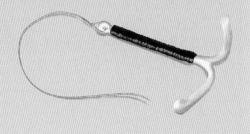

## Male condoms

✓ Offers significant protection against STDs if
   used correctly
✓ Widely available without needing access to
   a healthcare professional
✓ 98% effective in preventing pregnancy if
   used correctly

A condom is a thin sheath, usually made of
latex, that is rolled over a penis before sexual
intercourse. It works as a barrier to stop semen
from entering the vagina. Remember that with
all male condoms, withdrawal should happen
soon after ejaculation to avoid sperm leaking
into the vagina.

### Pros

If used correctly, condoms are 98 per cent
effective in preventing pregnancy. They
also significantly reduce your risk (and
your partner's risk) of contracting sexually
transmitted diseases. They are widely available
to purchase from pharmacies, supermarkets
and garages (as well as many bars and
restaurants) and can sometimes be obtained
free of charge from sexual health centres.
They also enable men to play an active part
in preventing pregnancy (instead of the onus
being on the woman) and, since they don't
require advance preparation, are an ideal way
to protect yourself during unplanned sexual
encounters. In most cases, condoms have no
medical side effects.

### Cons

You have to use a new condom each time you
have intercourse and, because they're not
generally available on prescription, this can
be expensive. Having to put it on the penis
before penetration means that sexual activity
can be disrupted, although many couples
happily incorporate it into their foreplay.
There's a risk that the condom will tear or slip
off during sex, so it's not the most failsafe
method of contraception.

Condoms made from latex are unsuitable
for anyone who's allergic to latex, but other
materials are available: polyisoprene condoms,
which are made from synthetic rubber
that is stretchy and provides a good fit; or
polyurethane condoms, which are made from
plastic rather than latex, so don't always fit very
snugly and can slip off. Lambskin, or 'natural',
condoms made from sheep intestines are also
available. These work to prevent pregnancy
but do not protect against STDs because the
material is porous and allows tiny viruses to
get through.

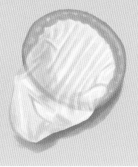

## Female condoms

✓ Offers good protection against STDs if used correctly

✓ Can be inserted long before sexual intercourse

✓ 95% effective in preventing pregnancy if used properly

Worn inside the woman's vagina, the female condom is made from thin latex and works by creating a barrier to prevent sperm reaching the uterus.

### Pros

Female condoms are available to buy from some pharmacies (and can be obtained from sexual health clinics) and, if used correctly, can offer good protection against STDs. Unlike the male version, the female condom can be inserted long before intercourse (so there's less interruption to sexual activity) and the man does not need to withdraw his penis immediately after ejaculation. There are no medical side effects, other than triggering allergic reactions to latex.

### Cons

Mastering the insertion technique can be tricky for many women, and the condom may feel a little uncomfortable when inside the vagina. If female condoms are used properly, they are 95 per cent effective, so are less reliable than other contraceptive methods. You need to use a new condom each time you have intercourse and, unlike the male version, they are not always widely available to buy on the high street. Female condoms made from latex are unsuitable for anyone who's allergic to latex.

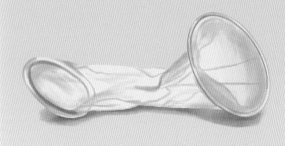

## Diaphragm

✓ Can be inserted up to two hours before sexual intercourse
✓ More environmentally friendly because it can be re-used for two years
✓ 92% effective in preventing pregnancy if used properly with spermicide
✗ Does not offer reliable protection against STDs

The diaphragm, also known as the cap, is a barrier method of contraception which is inserted into the vagina to fit over the cervix before sexual intercourse. It's usually used with spermicidal gel. There are different sizes available and you would usually be fitted for one by a healthcare profession (although there is now a one-size-fits-all diaphragm that can be purchased online, too). It needs to stay in place for at least six hours after sexual intercourse to be effective.

### Pros

Being a barrier method of contraception, it contains no hormones and will have no physical impact on your body (such as period disruption, breast tenderness, mood changes or low libido). The diaphragm gives the woman full control – it can be inserted up to two hours before sex – and, when washed after each use, one diaphragm can last for two years. Being so long lasting means it is the most environmentally friendly barrier method.

### Cons

This barrier method is not as effective as others. The one-size-fits-all diaphragm may be even less effective than a fitted diaphragm, with studies showing that, with *typical* use 17 out of 100 women will become pregnant after one year. Getting the diaphragm technique right can be tricky and fiddly; before you start using it, you'll need to make an appointment for a fitting with your doctor or nurse to double-check it's the right size and being put in the right place. You may need to be fitted for a new diaphragm or cap if you lose or gain more than 3kg in weight or have an abortion, and you should always be fitted for a new diaphragm after you have given birth.

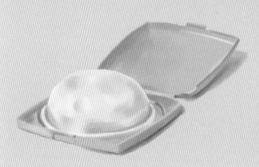

## Female sterilization

✓ Permanent, non-reversible option for people who do not want to ever be pregnant
✗ Does not provide protection against STDs

A tubal ligation is a minor surgical procedure that cuts or blocks the fallopian tubes. A hysterectomy is a more serious operation which removes the uterus (often carried out to treat conditions like uterine fibroids and pelvic pain). Both of these procedures are performed by a gynaecologist.

**Pros**
Both procedures are highly effective against pregnancy, since they offer permanent protection. They are options for someone who is certain they don't want to get pregnant, or does not want to have any more children. A hysterectomy will stop your periods, and will remove any risk of uterine or cervical cancer.

**Cons**
Tubal ligation may involve some pain. It does not affect your menstrual cycles and does not prevent any gynaecological cancers. A hysterectomy can have a very long recovery time. Both surgeries are non-reversible, and don't protect against STDs so you'll need to use a condom if you have multiple partners or a new partner.

## Withdrawal technique

✗ Not a reliable contraceptive option
✗ Does not provide protection against STDs
✓ 73% effective in preventing pregnancy

The withdrawal technique relies on a man withdrawing his penis from a woman's vagina before ejaculation. It is not a reliable contraceptive option but is sometimes used alongside period tracking to lessen the chance of pregnancy.

**Pros**
This is a natural, non-medical method with no cost implications. There are no physical or medical side effects, and it allows a man to play an active part in pregnancy prevention.

**Cons**
The withdrawal technique is not an effective method of contraception, primarily because it is difficult for a man to predict ejaculation, and the penis can leak some sperm in the prostatic fluid (pre-cum) before ejaculation. It has only a 73 per cent success rate, which means 27 out of 100 women using this withdrawal method for a year will become unintentionally pregnant. The associated worry about getting pregnant can decrease sexual pleasure for both parties and, without a barrier such as a condom, it doesn't protect against STDs.

## Emergency contraception

✓ The morning-after pill is at least 97% effective at preventing pregnancy if used properly (varies between brands)
✓ The IUD coil is over 99.9% effective at preventing pregnancy if fitted within five days of unprotected sex
✗ Does not provide protection against STDs
✗ Emergency contraception should not be used as your regular method

These are birth-control measures taken after you've had unprotected sex, in order to prevent pregnancy. Known as the morning-after pill, it works by preventing or delaying ovulation and, in order to maximize effectiveness, should be taken as soon as possible after unprotected sex. The morning-after pill is available over the counter from most pharmacies, and does not require a prescription. Some brands have to be taken within 72 hours (3 days) of sex, and others have to be taken within 120 hours (5 days) of sex. The IUD coil (see page 81) stops an egg from being fertilized or implanting in the uterus, and can be inserted into the uterus as an emergency intervention up to five days after unprotected sex, or up to five days after the earliest time the person could have ovulated.

### Pros

These methods are very effective at preventing pregnancy and you'll have a less than 0.1% chance of getting pregnant if the IUD coil is fitted within five days of unprotected sex, and a 3% chance if the morning-after pill is taken as directed.

### Cons

Morning-after pills are not effective if you vomit within three hours of taking them, so you may need another dose. They can also cause bloating, nausea and breast tenderness, and could make your menstrual cycle irregular. The IUD coil will need to be inserted at your doctor's surgery, and can be painful (see page 81). Neither of these methods protect against sexually transmitted diseases.

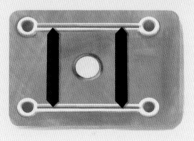

# Sexually transmitted diseases

Sexually transmitted diseases (also known as STDs or STIs – sexually transmitted infections) are a risk for anyone who has sexual intercourse or sexual contact with other people. It is vital that you know how to protect yourself from contracting them, and that you are aware of the early signs of STDs so that you can seek treatment.

Those who don't use barrier methods of contraception are particularly susceptible to STDs. Note that STDs can occur at any stage in your life, too, and – contrary to popular opinion – are not just restricted to people in their teens, twenties and thirties. I've definitely noticed an increase in older patients presenting with STD symptoms, particularly midlife women who – once their periods cease and their pregnancy risk abates – are choosing not to use condoms.

First and foremost, I'd advise anyone who's having sex to consider using barrier methods of contraception, even if you're on the Pill (and especially if you have a new partner or multiple partners). STDs can cause some really unpleasant symptoms yet can be easily avoided by taking a responsible approach to your own sexual health, and perhaps keeping a few condoms in your bag. It's also a good idea to familiarize yourself with your local sexual health clinic (sometimes called a genitourinary medicine or GUM clinic) should you ever need to visit it. Every area should have one of these specialist centres, which offers a range of confidential and non-judgemental services, including testing and treatment. They are usually accessed by making an appointment or by attending drop-in sessions (some clinics are aimed at specific groups, including young people and LGBTQ+ communities).

You should always book in for an STD screening if you notice any of the tell-tale symptoms, have had unprotected sex, have shared a needle or suffer an accidental needlestick injury. All STD centres have a secure and confidential contact-tracing system so they'll contact any current or former partners on your behalf.

You can also get any STD symptoms looked at by your doctor, if you prefer. And please don't feel embarrassed at the prospect of a clinician examining your genitals. We are so experienced in this field (I've seen thousands of vulvas and vaginas) and will always treat patients with the utmost care and respect.

Many STDs can be treated by antibiotics or antivirals, but you can catch them more than once, therefore practicing safe sex is vitally important.

These days, it's not uncommon for couples in the early stage of a relationship to get themselves checked out for STDs before they have sex (people in some local authority areas can receive free chlamydia, gonorrhoea and HIV self-testing kits delivered to their door). A trip to the GUM clinic may not be the most romantic date you'll ever go on, but it's one of the most responsible things you can do for each other.

I think it's really important that young people recognize the various STD symptoms. Granted, the following may not necessarily make pleasant reading, but it will help you spot the signs early and avoid future complications.

### The herpes virus

There are two types of herpes virus: type 1 herpes causes cold sores on the face, and type 2 causes sores on the genitals. The latter is a common STD that's passed on through sex (vaginal, oral or anal). An outbreak can cause small blisters around the genitals and is usually accompanied by a tingling, burning and itching sensation. These blisters can often burst open, exuding a clear liquid and leaving red open sores (women can also suffer vaginal discharge). The herpes virus can live in your body for years and then reappear, even if you've not had sex. There is no cure for it, but your doctor or STD clinic may be able to prescribe anti-viral medication to stop or reduce the severity of an outbreak.

### Chlamydia

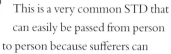

This is a very common STD that can easily be passed from person to person because sufferers can be symptom-free; indeed, some women only realize they have the infection years afterwards, when they have difficulty becoming pregnant. Those that do have symptoms often notice an unusual vaginal or penile discharge, pain on passing urine, pain when having sex, or pain in the abdominal area. Some women with chlamydia feel an ache when they're having a period. Chlamydia can be treated with antibiotics.

### Gonorrhoea

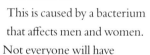

This is caused by a bacterium that affects men and women. Not everyone will have symptoms, but the key sign is a thick, yellow-green penile or vaginal discharge. Other symptoms include pelvic pain, pain while passing urine or stools, and bleeding during or after sex. Women can suffer bleeding between periods and, although rare, men can experience swollen testicles. Gonorrhoea can be treated with antibiotics.

### Trichomoniasis

This is caused by a parasite. It produces a yellow-green vaginal discharge that can be thick, thin or frothy, with a smelly, fishy odour. Other signs include genital soreness and itching, and pain while passing urine. Half of trichomoniasis sufferers have no symptoms, so it can be easily passed on. Trichomoniasis can be treated with antibiotics.

### Syphilis

This is caused by a bacterium, and symptoms might not always be obvious. They can include fever, fatigue, sore throat, aching joints, white patches in the mouth and swollen lymph nodes. Some people suffer a blotchy rash on the palms of the hands and the soles of the feet. Painless sores or ulcers around the vulva and anus can sometimes go unnoticed. Syphilis can be treated with antibiotics.

### Pubic lice

Also known as 'crabs', lice can cause itching around the pubic area. Some sufferers notice small white or pale-bluish spots around the genitals, thighs and lower abdominal area, and others can feel tired and run down. Pubic lice are treated by a malathion or permethrin lotion, which should be applied and left on for 12 hours then washed off. The treatment will need to be repeated seven days later to ensure that all the lice have been eradicated.

### Human papillomavirus (HPV)

This is in fact a group of around 100 different viruses, although not all are sexually transmitted. HPV is transmitted by genital skin contact, by vaginal, anal or oral sex, or by sharing sex toys. In most cases, men and women don't realize they have it, although a low-risk HPV may cause genital warts or an oral infection. A high-risk HPV may cause cell changes at the cervix that can cause cancer but this can be spotted and addressed during a routine cervical screening (otherwise known as a smear test – see page 153).

These tests are offered every three years to women aged between 25 and 49, and every five years to women aged between 50 and 64.

In the UK, all boys and girls born on or after 1 September 2006 are offered the HPV vaccine when they are aged between 12 and 13. The vaccine is offered to people up to 45 years old, but it's thought to be most effective when administered to a person before they become sexually active. Statistics in 2022 showed that HPV vaccines provided 87 per cent protection against cervical cancer.

### HIV (human immunodeficiency virus)

HIV is a sexually transmitted infection that can damage your immune system. Initial symptoms can be very vague, and can include weight loss, lack of energy, night sweats and recurrent infections. If HIV remains untreated, it can progress to a disease known as acquired immunodeficiency syndrome (AIDS).

HIV still remains a global issue, with no cure for the infection as such. However, thanks to huge advances in medical science, we now live in an age when HIV testing, diagnosis and treatment has become incredibly effective, so much so that the infection can be controlled by medication, and does not necessarily lead to AIDS. This wonderful development means that people with HIV are now able to live long and healthy lives. You can obtain an HIV test from your local sexual health clinic (it's free in some areas of the UK) or via charities such as the excellent Terrence Higgins Trust (see Resources from page 241).

# Considerations for trans individuals

In the following section, I shall largely use 'trans' as an umbrella term, but this refers to anyone with a uterus who defines themselves as transgender, non-binary or gender diverse.

The General Medical Council (GMC) states that 'trans and non-binary people experience the same health problems as everyone else, and have very few differing needs. If a health problem is related to gender identity, or its treatment, you must assess, provide treatment for and refer trans patients the same as you would other patients.'

Sadly, this guidance doesn't always apply in practice. For myriad reasons, many trans and non-binary people continue to suffer medical discrimination across the healthcare spectrum. This is something that needs to change, starting with more allies and advocates within surgeries and hospitals. As a GP, I'm committed to helping and supporting *all* patients, whether they happen to identify as cis gender, trans or otherwise.

Those assigned female at birth (AFAB) who no longer identify with that gender will require healthcare that's within my specialist remit and, like all my patients, will be treated with respect, and without bias. I am very conscious that I am often their first point of contact within a healthcare setting.

Much of the clinical guidance already outlined in this chapter will apply to a trans person who possesses a uterus. For example, I'll offer them the same advice about tracking their menstrual cycles, selecting appropriate contraception and monitoring their sexual health. They may well require treatment for issues such as endometriosis, premenstrual syndrome (PMS) or polycystic ovary syndrome (PCOS). However, I'm acutely aware that some trans people suffer with gender dysphoria, and will always take this into account.

According to the NHS, 'gender dysphoria is a term that describes a sense of unease that a person may have because their gender identity doesn't match their birth sex. This sense of unease or dissatisfaction may be so intense it can lead to depression and anxiety and have a harmful impact on daily life.'

Some trans people are fearful of (or repulsed by) their own anatomical features and characteristics, which can lead to feelings of anxiety and vulnerability during a clinical appointment or an examination. In these situations, I'll always do my very best to ease their worries and make them feel as comfortable as possible, which may include adopting different terminology, ensuring I use their preferred pronouns, or avoiding assumptions about their sexual preferences.

Trans men can present with distinct physiological and emotional needs and issues that may relate to the following areas.

## Menstruation

Monthly periods can be deeply problematic for a trans person suffering with dysphoria. If they wish to stop their menstrual cycle, we can discuss the suitability of long-term contraceptives, such as an implant or IUS coil. Younger patients, or perhaps those who've not had children, can be fitted with a more compact coil.

The contraceptive pill is another option. If a patient is not on testosterone therapy then they can be prescribed the combined contraceptive pill, which can be taken continuously for three months with a four-day break, reducing the number of periods they experience. If a patient is on testosterone therapy then they they can be prescribed the progesterone-only mini-pill, that can be taken continuously so they do not have periods. However, as the IUS and both contraceptive pills are hormonal treatments, consideration needs to be given to any other hormones a trans person might be prescribed as part of their gender affirmation therapy (such as testosterone).

## Fertility

If a trans patient with a uterus decides to embark on hormone treatment, yet still wishes to have biological children in the future, they may consider egg preservation; the Human Fertilisation and Embryology Authority (HFEA) website contains a wealth of information about this (see Resources from page 241).

Local Integrated Care Systems in England,Scotland and Wales should provide funding for fertility for trans patients and their policies should support *all* patients undergoing NHS treatment that is likely to affect their fertility.

## Mental health

Trans people are disproportionately affected by mental ill health that can be aggravated by the bigotry and prejudice they often face. Malicious misgendering, for example, or legal and social discrimination can exacerbate poor emotional wellbeing. The *Stonewall LGBT in Britain Health Report*, published in 2018, makes for disturbing reading. Results from a study group of 5,000 people found that 71 per cent of trans individuals had experienced anxiety during the previous year, with 35 per cent admitting to self-harm. Almost half of trans people (46 per cent) had experienced suicidal thoughts and 12 per cent had attempted to end their lives. I'm always mindful of these statistics, and I believe other clinicians should be, too. I really recommend the Stonewall website for further reading (see Resources from page 241).

## Eating disorders

Trans people, especially those suffering with dysphoria, can be particularly susceptible to eating disorders such as anorexia or bulimia (the Stonewall Report put the figure at 21 per cent, so that's roughly one in five). Being underweight can prompt the cessation or disruption of menstrual

*Your GP will signpost you to the specialist care and treatment you require. Ask the surgery receptionist which doctor is best placed to help you.*

periods, or can reduce the size of breasts, which is often the ulterior motive. Doctors like myself need to be aware of this and, if necessary, refer the patient for specialist support.

## Gender identity

At the time of writing, if you live in the UK, are 18 or over and are transgender, you can ask your doctor to refer you to a gender identity clinic, also known as a gender dysphoria clinic or GDC (see Resources from page 241 for more information). There, you'll receive specialist care that can range from psychological help to hormone therapy. With regard to the latter, trans women are typically prescribed oestrogen along with testosterone blockers, whereas trans men usually receive testosterone (and sometimes oestrogen blockers). Your GP will be kept in the loop by the GDC, and will be on hand to offer general practice-based support if you require it.

If you're under the age of 18 and are transgender, your family doctor can refer you to the Gender Identity Development Service (GIDS) that caters for the needs of children and young people. GPs will apply Gillick competence guidelines (see page 74) to any patient under the age of 16 who does not wish to involve their parents. The multidisciplinary team will offer you a wide range of services and resources, which may involve counselling and hormone therapy. As you approach adulthood, GIDS may refer you on to a Gender Identity Clinic where you can progress towards more permanent gender affirmation treatments. There is some useful information available online (see Resources from page 241).

## Chest binding

Chest binders are tight-fitting, elasticated vests that some trans men and non-binary people wear to flatten their breast tissue. The majority of these garments are made to strict specifications in order to meet safety standards, but it's often a good idea for a doctor to double-check that they're fitting properly. Overly tight binders can cause pain to the chest wall and ribs and can prevent sleep due to soreness. They can also cut into the skin, which may cause skin infections such as cellulitis. Even if you bind your chest, be sure to regularly examine the breast tissue for lumps (see pages 16–17).

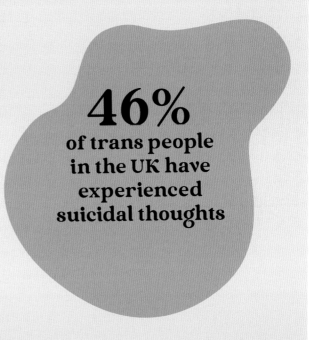

## 46%
### of trans people in the UK have experienced suicidal thoughts

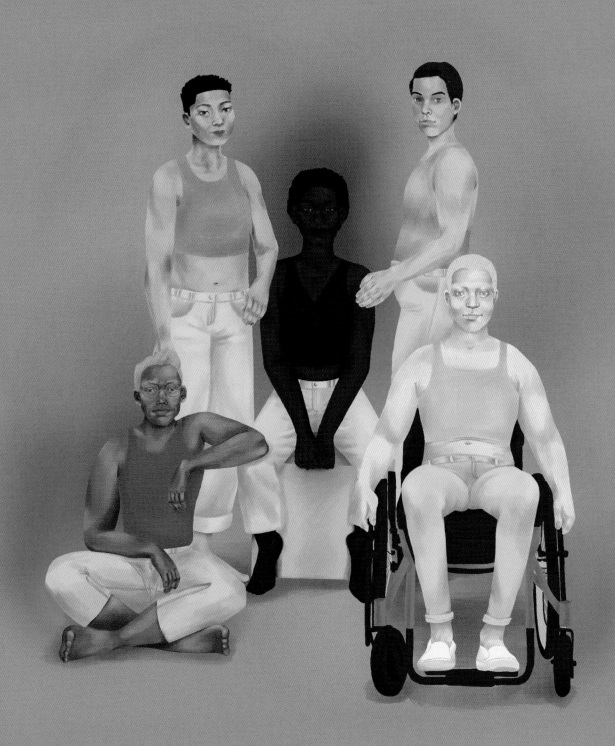

# Dr Nighat's Takeaways

## 1 See the doctor who's right for you

Make sure you register with your local healthcare provider and, if possible, ask to be seen by a clinician who specializes in women's or trans health.

## 2 Know your body and track your menstrual cycle

Download a period-tracking app onto your phone or note symptoms in a diary; it'll help you understand your monthly cycle (and your doctor will love you for it!).

## 3 Don't put up with period pain

Don't be a martyr to your pain! Paracetamol (and ibuprofen, if you can take it) can ease your symptoms and help you get on with life.

## 4 Weigh up your health options

Do your research, and choose the period products and contraceptive methods that best suit you. What's right for one person may not be right for another.

## 5 Share your views, concerns & expectations

Empower yourself – you're in charge! Outline your worries to your doctor, ask them lots of questions and discuss how your symptoms can be managed.

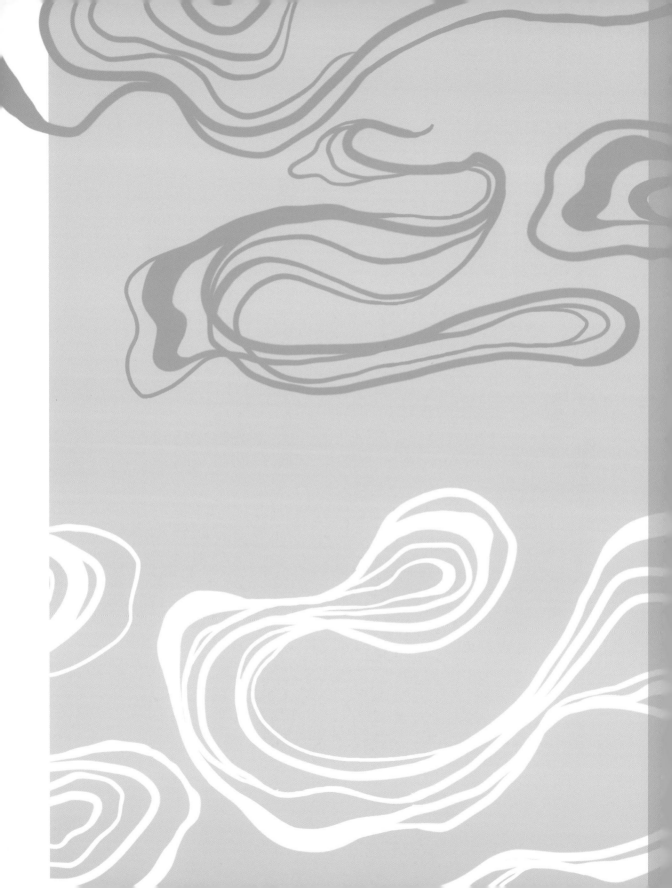

# Your Fertile Years

# Your fertile years: introduction

Planning for a baby can be one of the most thrilling times of your life. Introducing a little person into your household, along with all the love and happiness it will (hopefully) bring, can be a joyful prospect. So, if you've decided to take the plunge... many congratulations, and may I wish you all the luck in the world! ♥

Starting a family is such a momentous decision and, of course, there are lots of things to consider beforehand. 'Only have a baby when you're ready' is the advice I often give to my patients. Have a long, hard think about whether it's a sensible decision for all involved, and ask yourself a few important questions:

◆ Is it the right time for you to get pregnant?
◆ Are you in good health?
◆ Will you be able to juggle your home life with your work life?
◆ Can you afford childcare?
◆ Do you have a decent support network?
◆ Is your relationship in a good place?

Indeed, if you do have a partner, please ensure that you're both ready and willing to go down this route. I've faced awkward situations in my surgery when one half of the couple isn't sold on the idea of having a baby, unbeknownst to the other. I remember one patient whispering to me that they were secretly using contraception as they weren't ready for the patter of tiny feet!

As for timing your pregnancy, it's commonly known that your best reproductive years from a biological standpoint are in your twenties, when your ovaries store the highest number of good-quality eggs, and when your pregnancy risks are at their lowest.

Fertility begins to decline gradually during your thirties – particularly after the age of 35 – but that doesn't mean you can't become pregnant during that time or beyond. Depending on lifestyle and other factors, there's no reason why women in their thirties, maybe up to their mid-forties, can't go on to give birth to healthy babies.

However, as someone who's dealt with all manner of fertility and pregnancy-related issues – and as a mother of three myself – I've learned you have to start managing your expectations. Despite your best efforts and intentions, you cannot schedule in a baby. Like buses, they'll come when they want to (and sometimes it can be two or three at once!). The journey towards pregnancy can be erratic and unpredictable and you may have to prepare yourself for lots of twists, turns and bumps in the road. Things may not always go quite to plan, and the whole process can often be fraught with stress, worry and confusion.

Prospective parents who come to my surgery always have lots of questions – rightly so; it's a life-changing decision – and I hope this part of the book provides you with a few answers, as well as some useful tips and advice.

In this chapter I'll be looking at fertility and pregnancy issues through a family doctor's lens, which means I'll be outlining the most common cases and conditions we face in general practice. More specific issues that might ordinarily be addressed by your midwife, gynaecologist or obstetrician, therefore, may not be covered in depth. With this in mind, check out the Resources section to help you find excellent sources of information about the second and third pregnancy trimesters, as well as the birth itself.

This section of the book will largely refer to male and female partnerships, but I'm mindful that families come in all configurations. Indeed, some of the happiest, healthiest and well-cared-for children who visit my surgery belong to single-parent families, or belong to parents from the LGBTQ+ community. These people should receive the same level of care and support as anybody else, of course, so much of my advice will apply to them. The NHS offers information for transgender and non-binary pregnant people and other health authorities should too (see Resources from page 241).

Towards the end of this section I'll also be covering other health considerations that people of child-bearing age need to be aware of, such as health screening and recognizing symptoms of gynaecological cancer.

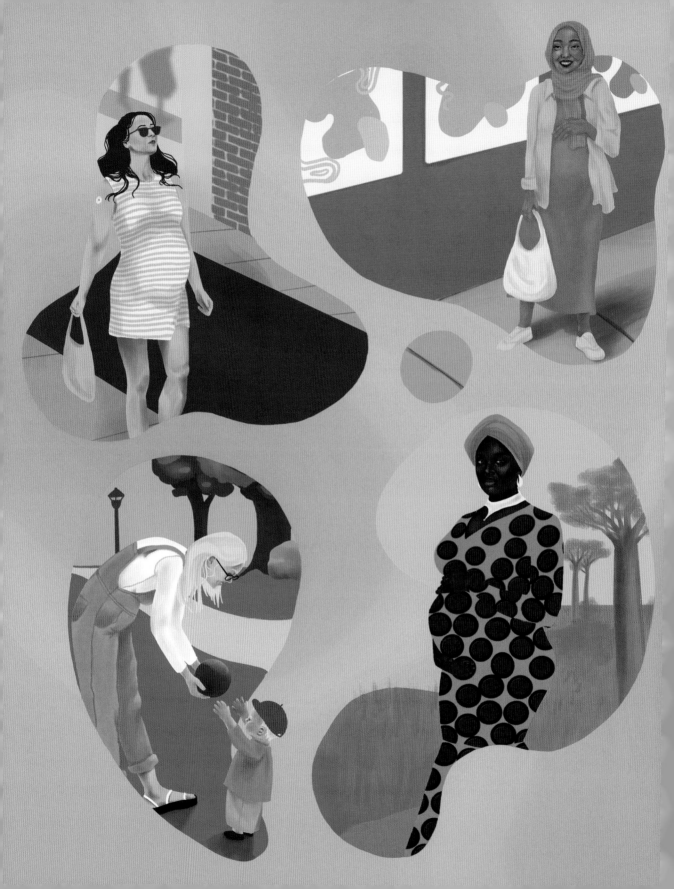

# Planning for pregnancy

If you've set your heart on becoming pregnant, my advice is to plan ahead, gather as much information as you can and get yourself in the best possible shape. If you're in a relationship, the latter applies to your partner, too – the fitter and healthier you both are, the more likely you'll conceive. Ideally, you should try to make the following changes to your health and lifestyle.

## Dietary supplements & lifestyle changes

It is important to ensure your baby gets adequate nutrients from the point of conception. A healthy, varied diet should be complemented by nutritional supplements and a healthy lifestyle.

### Take folic acid

Folic acid reduces the baby's chances of having neural tube defects (NTDs) such as spina bifida. One to three months before you begin trying to conceive you should take 400 micrograms (0.4 milligrams) of folic acid every day, and for at least 12 weeks after conception. Current recommendations actually advise women to continue taking it throughout pregnancy and during breastfeeding, too. You may take 5,000 micrograms (5.0 milligrams) of folic acid if you or the other biological parent has a neural tube defect, if you've previously had a pregnancy affected by an NTD, have diabetes, or you or your partner takes anti-epilepsy medication.

### Take vitamins

All pregnant individuals should take 10 micrograms (400iu) of vitamin D throughout their pregnancy and while breastfeeding. However, be careful to avoid multivitamins that contain vitamin A (retinol), as too much of this in the first trimester can harm the baby's development by affecting the nervous and cardiovascular systems and, in rare cases, trigger spontaneous miscarriage. It is also advisable to avoid liver and liver products (including fish liver oil) during this time as they contain high levels of vitamin A.

### Stop smoking

Smoking cigarettes during pregnancy is linked to miscarriage, high levels of premature birth, low birth weight and sudden infant death syndrome (SIDS). The baby also has an increased chance of having breathing problems in the first six months of life. Quitting the habit can be hard, I know, but it's the sensible thing to do for you and your baby. Luckily, there is so much support out there, including the free NHS Quit Smoking app that you can download onto your phone (see Resources from page 241). The app allows you to track your progress, offers you motivational support, and even shows you how much money you're saving. According to NHS data, if you can make it to 28 days without smoking, you're five times more likely to quit for good!

### Stop drinking

Alcohol guidance for pregnant women has changed a great deal over the years. Gone are the days when you were encouraged to drink a famous Irish stout! As it stands, current guidance recommends that alcohol should be completely avoided, since it increases the risk of miscarriage, premature birth and low birth weight. Drinking heavily during pregnancy may also cause your baby to develop foetal alcohol spectrum disorder (FASD), a serious condition that can lead to lifelong issues.

Judging by those who visit my surgery, the vast majority choose to stick to a no-alcohol rule while they're pregnant. I know some women find it hard to kick the 'wine o'clock' habit, but there are many great alcohol-free drinks available to try. My personal favourites include alcohol-free gin with tonic and zero-alcohol beer (fab with a curry!).

### Review your medications

Always check with your doctor that any medication you have been prescribed is safe to take during pregnancy. There has been some controversy surrounding sodium valproate, a drug that treats conditions such as epilepsy and bipolar disorder, since it's said to have caused birth defects and developmental problems. As far as I'm concerned, this medication should *never* be prescribed to women of child-bearing age but, in the event that it is, it should only be given to those taking contraceptives. Don't hesitate to raise any concerns about sodium valproate with your doctor.

### Avoid recreational drugs

You must stop using recreational drugs such as cocaine and cannabis, both before and after your pregnancy. Substance and/or alcohol abuse can affect a parent's ability to look after their child,

and can cause real danger if they fall asleep next to an infant (there have been tragic cases of babies being accidentally suffocated when a drowsy parent rolls over in the middle of the night).

### Stick to a healthy weight

It's always very sensible to keep to a healthy weight, whatever stage of life you're at, but this is particularly important if you're trying to conceive.

If you're overweight with a BMI (body mass index) above 30, you may have issues conceiving or responding to fertility treatment. You also have an increased risk of miscarriage (see page 115), high blood pressure, deep vein thrombosis (DVT) and gestational diabetes (see page 119). Before you become pregnant, I advise you to use a BMI calculator to keep track of your weight and also to consider using a health and fitness app or website. There are some brilliant options out there, many available for free (see Resources from page 241).

To calculate your body mass index, divide your weight in kilograms by your height in metres squared (or use an online calculator!)
BMI = $kg/m^2$.

If you're underweight with a BMI below 18.5, you may be more likely to experience hormonal imbalances that could affect ovulation and may affect your chances of getting pregnant. I have many underweight patients who go on to have healthy babies, but having a low BMI can put you at a higher risk of miscarriage, and can increase your chances of having a premature birth (when the baby is born before it is fully developed), an underweight baby, or a baby that suffers with gastroschisis (a condition whereby the baby's stomach does not develop properly).

If you have an underlying eating disorder that may be contributing to your low weight, please talk to your doctor about arranging a prenatal assessment. There is also a great deal of practical support available from charities and other organizations (see Resources from page 241).

### Check your vaccinations

It's vital to ensure that you're up to date with your vaccinations. Having your MMR (measles, mumps and rubella) jab is particularly important, because rubella – commonly known as German measles – can harm your baby if you contract it while pregnant, particularly in the early stages. If you're unsure about your immunization history, speak to your health practitioner who will be able to access your medical records or carry out a blood test to check your rubella immunity. And, if you're given the MMR jab, you should avoid becoming pregnant within one month of the vaccine.

One of the most common questions I'm asked by pregnant people is, 'Should I have the Covid-19 vaccination?' My answer is a categorical *yes*. In April 2021, the RCOG (Royal College of Obstetricians and Gynaecologists) and the JCVI (Joint Committee on Vaccination and Immunization) concluded that the Covid-19 jab was safe and could be given at any time during pregnancy, but preferably after the first trimester. I firmly believe that if you're offered the vaccine, you should take it, as pregnant women who contract Covid-19 are more likely to have complications from it (although they are at no greater risk of being infected in the first place). Data shows that one in five pregnant women who have become unwell with the virus give birth early so, by having the vaccine, mums-to-be will be safeguarding themselves from going into premature labour. Not only that, the vaccine also provides immunity to the baby against Covid-19.

### Underlying conditions

If you have one of the following long-term underlying conditions, you'll be put under the care of a specialist consultant obstetrician for the duration of your pregnancy, alongside your midwife care, as your pregnancy will be considered higher risk:

- Diabetes
- High blood pressure
- A heart condition (or previous heart condition)
- Thyroid issues
- Cancer
- Mental health conditions

Routinely, anyone with Afro-Caribbean, Mediterranean, Indian, Pakistani, Southeast Asian and Middle Eastern heritage should be offered a screening test for two inherited blood disorders – sickle cell disease and thalassemia. You can also ask for a free test from your doctor if you're worried you might be predisposed to these conditions.

### Sexually transmitted diseases

Depending on your sexual history – whether you've had unprotected sex, for example – you and your partner may want to book yourselves in for an STD review before you begin trying for a baby. You can make an appointment at your local sexual health clinic where you'll be tested and treated for free, with the utmost confidentiality.

When left untreated, some STDs can affect you and the developing baby – a gonorrhoea infection (see page 88), for example, can lead to miscarriage, premature birth, low birth weight and chorioamnionitis (a bacterial infection of the membranes that surround the foetus and the amniotic fluid in which the baby floats). Gonorrhoea can also affect the baby as it passes through the birth canal and, if left untreated, can cause eye infections in the child.

STDs can also cause scarring and blockage of the male and female reproductive structures. If they remain untreated in women, this can lead to an episode of pelvic inflammatory disease (PID, see page 144), which is a leading cause of infertility.

## Increasing your chances of conceiving

Conception is such an inexact science. It's impossible to say how long it will take a woman to become pregnant, because so much depends on the circumstances of each individual and each couple. The fortunate among us will become pregnant straight away, while others will take longer or, very sadly, will never be able to conceive by 'natural' methods. According to NHS figures, 92 per cent of women aged between 19 and 26 will conceive within one year, and 98 per cent will conceive within two years. If you're aged between 35 and 39, 82 per cent will conceive within one year and 90 per cent within two years.

However, in order to maximize your chances of conceiving, I'd suggest, in the first instance, you should follow the tips on planning for pregnancy I've outlined above. Once all that's in place, it's time for the fun bit! Having regular sexual intercourse is an essential part of conception, of course, particularly around the time that the woman is ovulating (releasing an egg). There are a number of ways you can monitor this:

- **Track your cycle** using an app or a diary (ovulation occurs about 14 days after your period starts).
- **Record your body temperature** with a thermometer (it rises up to a degree during ovulation).
- **Use an ovulation test kit** (this detects any increase in the luteinizing hormone in your urine).
- **Keep an eye on your normal vaginal mucus** (it might be wetter, clearer or more 'slippery' at the time of ovulation).
- **Take note of any breast tenderness**, breast swelling, abdominal pain or bloating (these can also be signs of ovulation, but working it out this way is not always that accurate).

The National Institute for Health and Care Excellence (NICE) guidance suggests you should have good-quality vaginal sex (with ejaculation) with your partner every two or three days, without contraception. Contrary to popular belief, daily intercourse isn't always a good idea because it can lead to a decrease in sperm concentration. And, forgive me for stating the obvious, but always ensure the sperm enters the vagina!

## Fertility problems

Statistically, one in seven couples will experience fertility related problems that create an obstacle to achieving parenthood. If you've not conceived successfully after one year of unprotected sex, on average, there may be an underlying problem that needs further investigation. Having problems conceiving is a very normal occurrence, but this doesn't make it any less distressing. You may think you've ticked all the boxes – having regular sex, following a healthy lifestyle – yet that dreaded period keeps arriving every month, like an unwelcome visitor. In these circumstances, there's no harm in visiting your doctor to talk things through and assess your situation. If you're in a relationship, I think it's really important to address these issues together. Emotions can run high on both sides – there's often a lot of guilt, anxiety and frustration – but, in order to reach your goal, you and your partner will need to support one another. It takes two to make a baby, after all.

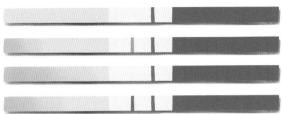

Ovulation tests are useful to show your most-fertile window each month. Similar to a pregnancy test, they show two lines – a control and a test line – when you are ovulating.

Society still places blame at the woman's feet, but it's understood that 50 per cent of cases are specifically related to male fertility problems (usually the result of a low sperm count). Other fertility problems could be associated with at least one of these factors:

- Age
- Sexual intercourse quality or frequency; regular sex means unprotected vaginal sex at least every two to three days.
- Physical disorders: obesity, anorexia, breathing problems, cardiovascular issues.
- Sexually transmitted diseases (STDs).
- Hormonal problems such as polycystic ovary syndrome (PCOS), early menopause and issues with thyroid or pituitary glands.
- Reproductive system problems, such as pelvic inflammatory disease (PID), blocked fallopian tubes, adenomyosis and endometriosis.

It's the latter two issues – hormonal and reproductive system complications – that I'd like to focus on here. I see many patients in my surgery whose fertility is affected by these problems, and I'm keen to do all I can to raise awareness.

# 1 in 7
## couples in the UK are affected by infertility

# Infertility (& your options)

Around one in seven couples are unable to conceive naturally. Sometimes this is due to known hormonal or reproductive issues but sometimes – despite a succession of tests, scans and examinations – the problem remains unexplained.

If you and your partner are healthy, having unprotected sex and have been unable to conceive a child after trying for one year, you should both see your doctor. They will discuss possible ways forward with you, and will outline a number of options. The good news is that many infertile people *can* go on to become parents. Thanks to the wonders of modern medicine and specialist intervention, up to 80 per cent of couples (or single parents) are able to have children.

## Getting the basics right

Healthy lifestyle habits will help create optimum conditions, and it's important to remember that these should apply to *both* potential parents, as sperm quality and quantity can be harmed by an unhealthy lifestyle.

- **Try to keep to a healthy weight** – have plenty of exercise and ensure you have a good diet. Sometimes it's helpful to have a prenatal discussion with your doctor to look at weight reduction (or weight gain).
- **Cut out smoking** as there are absolutely no benefits!
- **Cut down alcohol** consumption as much as possible.
- **Have regular unprotected sex** at least twice a week.
- **Manage your anxiety and stress**; trying to get pregnant can be an anxious time as a couple, so you might consider cognitive behavioural therapy (CBT).
- **Keep track of your ovulation window** using a luteinizing hormone kit.

## Getting help if you're having difficulty becoming pregnant

Firstly, book an appointment with your family doctor. Most appointments are only ten minutes long, so try to book a double (20-minute) appointment for you and your partner. During this appointment, your doctor will discuss your situation and medical history. This may include questions about your lifestyle, but may also include some very intimate questions about your sexual and gynaecological history.

The doctor might also perform a physical examination, perhaps a bi-manual exam for the female (sometimes using a plastic speculum) and a testicular examination for the male. Your doctor may also order the following tests:

- Baseline health check for both partners.
- Full blood count.
- Kidney, thyroid and liver function.
- Cholesterol check and diabetes check.
- Chlamydia test.
- Progesterone/gonadotropins check (female partner).
- A referral for a transvaginal ultrasound scan of the uterus, ovaries and fallopian tubes (female partner).
- A sperm analysis (male partner).

## Medical procedures to improve female fertility

Following your doctor's initial investigations, you will be referred directly to a hospital's obstetrics and gynaecology department in order to establish the underlying reason for infertility. From then on, family doctors will not prescribe or instigate any fertility medications themselves, but we will often have conversations with our patients about the various options they might be offered by their hospital consultant.

Medical options to improve female fertility include the following medications:

- **Metformin**, which is used in women with PCOS to help with insulin resistance and assist weight loss.
- **Clomifene citrate (clomid)**, which can help to regulate ovulation in women who have irregular periods.
- **Gonadotropins**, which can help to stimulate ovulation, and also help with male infertility.

These medications can have side effects, and giving ovulation-stimulating drugs to couples with unexplained infertility is not recommended unless under specialist guidance.

## Surgical procedures to improve female fertility

Once you've been assessed, if the issues affecting your fertility have been identified, you may be referred for surgical procedures to correct the issue. Surgical procedures to improve female fertility include the following:

- **Fallopian tube surgery** can be performed to correct any blockages or scarring found in the fallopian tubes. The success of the surgery depends on the extent of the blockage or scarring in the tubes.

- **Laparoscopic surgery** investigates whether endometriosis or PCOS is affecting your chances of getting pregnant. If there is endometriosis, and adhesions are noticed, then adhesiolysis (cutting away of the lesions) can help with pain and can assist with pregnancy (see page 140).
- **Ovarian drilling** is a laparoscopic surgical procedure that involves drilling away the ovarian cysts that have formed as a result of PCOS; this can help when ovulation-stimulating medication has not.

## Assisted conception

Assisted conception refers to a range of specialist treatments, including intra-uterine insemination (IUI) and in-vitro fertilization (IVF), that can help a patient to get pregnant. If my patients are interested in obtaining fertility treatments on the NHS, I'll suggest they read the relevant NICE guidelines as the availability of IUI and IVF is dependent on the funding of your local Integrated Care Boards (ICBs). These tend to follow the criteria below and are usually only available to couples who do not already have children:

- Three IVF cycles for women who are under the age of 40, and who've been trying for two years.
- One IVF cycle for women who are aged between 40 and 42.

The main assisted conception options for those in heterosexual relationships who are struggling to become pregnant, same-sex couples or those who wish to start a single-parent family, are listed below:

- **Intra-uterine insemination (IUI)** is the procedure whereby sperm is directly placed into the uterus (this could be your partner's sperm or donated sperm). This may take place if vaginal intercourse is not possible, or may be an option for same-sex couples. Ordinarily, same-sex couples can have six cycles of IUI and, if they don't become pregnant, will need to look at private options. Indeed, some couples pay for their treatment anyway because NHS waiting times for IUI are extremely long.

◆ **In-vitro fertilization (IVF)** is a process in which the egg is fertilized with sperm in a laboratory and then placed into the uterus. The egg and sperm can belong to the couple, or can be donated. The process of IVF is extremely intense and may not always be successful – younger women are more likely to have a successful assisted pregnancy, and IVF is not recommended by the NHS for women older than 42 (for that reason, many decide to seek private treatment). I always advise my patients to try to remain positive, but also to prepare themselves for a lot of stress and anxiety (and financial hardship). Getting the right advice and support is crucial, as is doing your research. See Resources from page 241 for more information.

There are six stages of IVF:

1 Suppression of natural menstrual cycle, involving daily medication to stop the normal cycle and expel the uterus lining.

2 Stimulation of ovulation, involving daily medication to encourage extra eggs to be released by the ovaries. During stimulation, ultrasound scans are performed every 1–3 days to check the progress of the maturation of the eggs.

3 Preparation for egg collection, involving a single dose of human chorionic gonatrophin (hCG) medication given at a precise time once scans show the eggs are ready for collection. You will be given an exact time for your egg collection in the next 24 hours.

4 Egg collection, a procedure during which a long, thin needle is put into the vagina and the eggs are harvested from the lining of the uterus.

5 Fertilization, a process when the retrieved eggs are mixed with the sperm in a laboratory test tube for a few days to allow fertilization.

6 Transfer of embryo: the fertilized embryos are placed back in the uterus. Usually you will be asked to wait two weeks before taking a pregnancy test.

## Other considerations

There are a number of other areas of fertility treatment and help that can be used alongside IVF and IUI. These include:

◆ **Egg/sperm donation**, which involves someone donating their eggs or sperm to people who are unable to use their own to become pregnant. If you have female- or male-factor infertility you may find donated eggs or sperm will help you. I would always advise patients to use a licensed clinic where the sperm and eggs are carefully screened for sexually transmitted diseases and/or genetic disorders. Reputable clinics will also provide appropriate legal advice to their clients. Alternatively, you may wish to donate yourself. Helping others in this way is such a wonderful, selfless thing to do, and there are now many NHS schemes that allow people to donate.

◆ **Egg preservation/egg harvesting/egg freezing** is a method that takes unfertilized eggs from the ovaries and freezes them, preserving them for future use.

## Alternative routes to parenthood

Medical and surgical procedures aren't suitable, or successful, for everyone. Many people become parents by surrogacy or adoption, while others may choose to become foster carers. Living child-free – out of choice or circumstance – is a perfectly reasonable alternative, too.

# Your body has not failed you because you didn't fall pregnant 'naturally'.

# LGBTQ+ parents & assisted conception

More and more members of the LGBTQ+ community are choosing to become parents these days. Society has changed, thank goodness – hooray for diversity and equality! – and families now come in all shapes and sizes. Anyone who wants to have children should of course receive the same care and consideration from healthcare professionals, regardless of their sexual preference or gender identity.

Many lesbian couples (or single people) I see in my surgery choose to conceive via sperm donor insemination and – if they encounter fertility problems – should have the same access to medical or surgical interventions (such as IVF) as detailed on pages 106–8. In the UK, there are some fairly complex legal implications to consider regarding donor insemination, though – mostly relating to parental rights and civil partnerships – about which more information can be found on websites listed in the Resources section from page 241.

If a trans person assigned female at birth (AFAB) is considering gender reassignment – with hormonal treatment and/or surgical transition – they may wish to preserve their fertility beforehand. Egg harvesting (see page 108) would be the usual option in these circumstances.

## Adoption & foster caring

LGBTQ+ people have had the same rights to adopt a child or become foster carers as other parents since 2005 in the UK and the number of families with same-sex parents is growing every year. Potential single parents should also not be discriminated against if they wish to adopt or become a foster carer either. This option can make a hugely valuable contribution to your community, and change a child's life.

# 1 in 6
## adoptions in England in 2021 were to same-sex couples

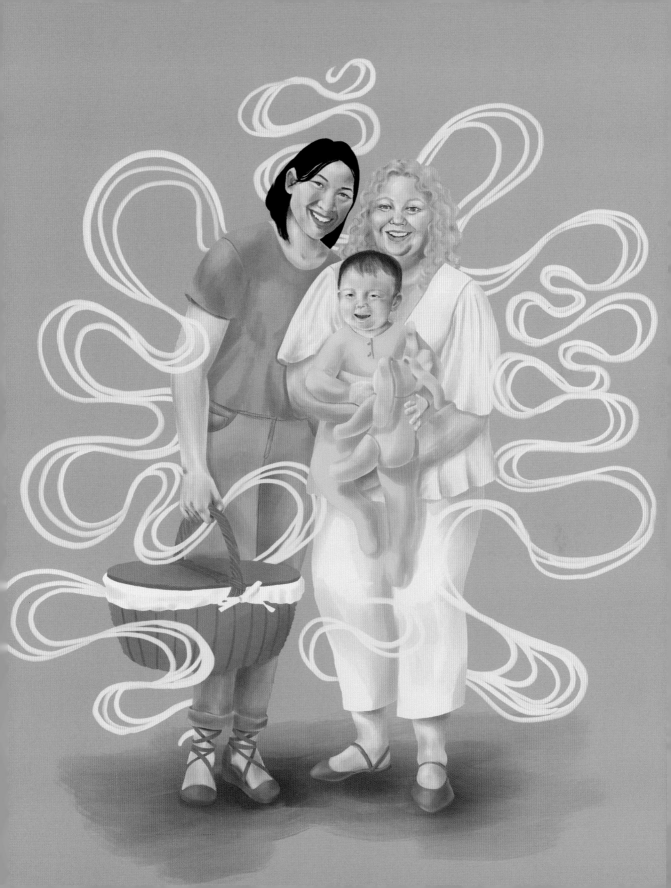

# IMPORTANT!
Do not let other people pressure or coerce you into doing something against your will. It is your body, and your decision.

Choose the right option for you.

# Testing for pregnancy

You can buy a pregnancy test over-the-counter from your local pharmacy or supermarket, and they are also available at sexual health clinics. Most tests are more than 99 per cent accurate.

You can take a pregnancy test from the first day of a missed period. Doing one before that time isn't advisable since the level of the pregnancy hormone (human chorionic gonadotropin, or hCG) may be too low to show up on a test and might give a negative result even if you are pregnant. If you have an irregular cycle and are unsure about the timing of your period, the earliest time to take a test is three weeks after you've had unprotected sex.

Before you confirm things with a test, however, you may already have a suspicion that you're pregnant. A missed menstrual period is the most obvious sign, but other tell-tale symptoms can include tender, swollen breasts, a change in mood, and nausea (with or without vomiting).

## Getting a positive pregnancy test result if you've planned a baby

Depending on your circumstances, receiving a positive pregnancy test may evoke a wide range of emotions. If you've planned to have a baby, you'll no doubt be walking on air and feeling hugely excited at this new chapter. As the reality sinks in, though, you may start to experience some less than positive feelings. A few of my patients worry they've made the wrong decision, and others become fearful about the act of giving birth. These are perfectly normal and natural responses, and there's no shame in discussing how you feel with your loved ones or a healthcare professional.

Once you've processed your good news, and are sure you want to go ahead with the pregnancy, you need to contact your healthcare provider to make a midwife assessment appointment (sometimes called the 'booking in' appointment). Here, you'll receive all the necessary antenatal advice, will be referred to your local hospital's maternity services, and will be listed for all the requisite scans and screenings. You'll receive a blood test at this appointment, too.

In reality, most GPs have little involvement with a person during their nine months of pregnancy, particularly if they are in good health with no associated complications. It's safer and more cost-effective for care to be offered by midwives, and nowadays, a pregnant person has a lot of autonomy and control in this important phase in their life. They'll be given their own maternity health record, which will contain all the notes from the midwife, the family doctor, the hospital team, the sonographer and anyone else that might need to be involved (dietician, physiotherapist, social services, and so on). It is a really useful communication tool.

A positive pregnancy test will show two lines: control line and test line (see top test). A negative pregnancy test will just show the control line (see bottom test).

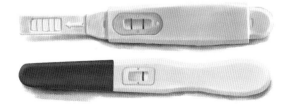

As a GP, I rarely have input in a patient's pregnancy, but will occasionally be contacted by a community midwife who may need specific advice or information, or by a consultant obstetrician if someone under their care requires prescribed medication. Other than that, the next time I see my patient they're often sitting in my surgery with a bouncing baby on their knee!

## Getting a positive pregnancy test result if you've not planned a baby

If your positive pregnancy test is unexpected, you may feel lots of different emotions. Firstly, try not to panic; unexpected pregnancies can happen to the best of us. Once you've got over the shock you will, of course, have to assess your options and decide how you wish to proceed. In order to help you with this, I'd urge you to talk things through with your partner, a trusted friend or family member, someone well placed to give you sensible, rational advice. But if you feel you can't talk to a loved one, you can book an appointment with your doctor or practice nurse, either of whom will treat you with care and sensitivity and will offer you informed and non-judgemental advice. There is also a wealth of advice available from charities and other organizations, too (see Resources from page 241).

### Continuing with a pregnancy

Should you decide to go ahead with the pregnancy, the procedure on page 113 will apply. Some people may choose to continue with the pregnancy but have their baby adopted after the birth; this process would ordinarily be looked after by a local authority's social services department and/or an adoption agency.

### Ending a pregnancy

If you live in England, Wales or Scotland and decide to terminate the pregnancy before 24 weeks, please make an appointment as soon as possible with your doctor, sexual health clinic or the British Pregnancy Advice Service (BPAS). A clinician will advise you and counsel you, without judgement or prejudice, and will refer you to an abortion clinic for further assessment and treatment. After 24 weeks, a termination can only be performed under extreme circumstances, for example if the mother's life is at risk or the child is likely to be born with severe disability.

You may also refer yourself to a private abortion clinic, where you'll have to pay for the procedure (the costs vary). Your local NHS sexual health clinic will have details of nearby services.

If you are under 16, your parents do not need to be told you are planning a termination, but you may be encouraged (but not pressured) to confide in a loved one for physical and mental support. Sometimes a family doctor will refer a patient to another colleague in the surgery if they are unable to participate in abortion for religious or ethical reasons. Ending a pregnancy can be a traumatic experience that necessitates lots of help and support. See Resources from page 241 for organizations that offer advice and guidance.

The abortion law in Northern Ireland changed in March 2020. Women currently have access to a termination up until 12 weeks gestation (that is, 11 weeks and 6 days) without any conditions, and from 12 to 24 weeks if the pregnancy is impacting the woman's physical or mental health. Please consult the Resources section from page 241 for the most up-to-date guidelines.

# Early pregnancy issues

In general practice, if a patient experiences early pregnancy bleeding (about 20 per cent of women have some bleeding in the first 12 weeks of pregnancy) or any other associated complications, I immediately refer them to our local early pregnancy unit for an ultrasound scan. From that point on they'll be looked after by the midwife and the obstetrician who will update me on their condition. If the patient sadly suffers baby loss, I will contact them to offer my condolences and will signpost them for support (see Resources on page 241).

## Miscarriage

Sadly, around one in every eight known pregnancies will end in miscarriage. Vaginal bleeding is the main sign, but light bleeding can be common in early pregnancy anyway. Always seek medical advice if you experience bleeding. Miscarriages can also occur without bleeding and are usually identified when your first pregnancy scan reveals the baby has no heartbeat. This is known as a missed miscarriage. After a miscarriage, the tissue of the pregnancy may pass out of your body naturally, or you may be given medicine or a surgical procedure to remove any remaining pregnancy tissue.

The majority of miscarriages occur in the first trimester. It is not usually possible to identify the exact cause, but miscarriages are rarely caused by something that you have done. It is believed that most early pregnancy loss is caused by abnormal chromosomes in the baby. Less commonly (one in four miscarriages), miscarriages can occur in the second trimester.

A miscarriage can be extremely distressing. Look after yourself physically and emotionally. You will be referred to an early pregnancy unit and your doctor will be able to connect you with counselling services if you require them. And

please remember that most miscarriages are one-off occurrences and can often be followed by a healthy pregnancy, if that is your wish.

## Ectopic pregnancy

One in eighty women will suffer an ectopic pregnancy, when the fertilized egg (ovum) gets stuck somewhere outside the uterus. Common symptoms include:

- Acute or dull pain in the lower abdomen.
- Unusual vaginal bleeding.
- Feeling faint, or collapsing.
- Nausea and vomiting, or loss of appetite.
- Bowel or bladder problems.
- Breast pain.
- Delayed periods.
- Pain during sex.

An ectopic pregnancy is a medical emergency, so if you are pregnant and suspect this may be happening you must go to straight to A&E for urgent scanning and assessment. Do not visit your family doctor, as this will only delay matters.

If you are experiencing these symptoms but have had a negative pregnancy test, particularly one that you think may be inaccurate – you must still flag this up to a clinician. Go straight to hospital. It could save your life.

## Possible ectopic pregnancy sites

An ectopic pregnancy occurs when the fertilized egg (ovum) becomes stuck outside the uterus. This diagram highlights where an ectopic pregnancy can occur. On rare occasions, two pregnancies can occur that result in ectopic pregnancies. A heterotopic pregnancy is when two embryos are present in different places of the reproductive system and a twin ectopic pregnancy is when two embryos are stuck in the same place.

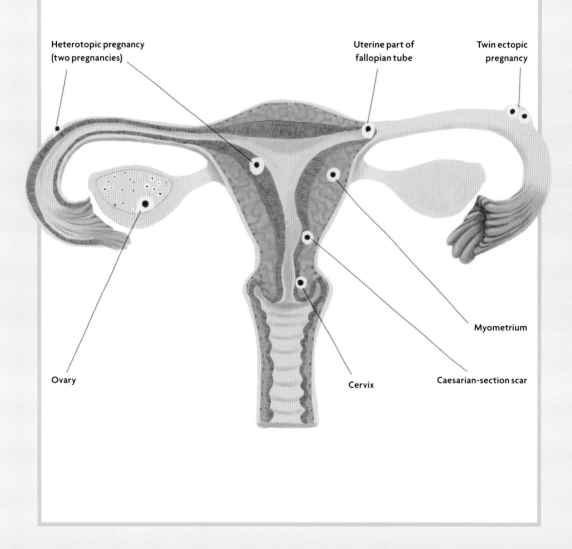

Heterotopic pregnancy (two pregnancies)

Uterine part of fallopian tube

Twin ectopic pregnancy

Myometrium

Ovary

Cervix

Caesarian-section scar

# Your body during pregnancy

Pregnancy is divided into three parts, know as trimesters, and during these trimesters your body is undertaking an incredible task – converting a bundle of cells into a living baby over a period of nine months (or 40 weeks). These months are not without their side effects, however, and many women can feel quite unwell at times during their pregnancy. The following pages are a guide of common pregnancy symptoms and those that warrant further attention from your doctor or pregnancy care team.

Many pregnant women find the first trimester particularly exhausting, something that is exacerbated by the fact that they often do not make their pregnancy public knowledge until after the first trimester is finished! The following areas of symptoms can be very common in pregnancy and shouldn't be cause for alarm. Please try to give yourself plenty of time to relax and acknowledge that you may need to take it easier over these next few months. As always, trust your instinct, and if you feel like any of these issues are particularly debilitating, then seek medical advice:

## Common effects of pregnancy

- **Nausea & vomiting** is particularly common in the first trimester of pregnancy, but can ease off by weeks 16 to 20. Unfortunately, some women find they are nauseous all the way through pregnancy. Make sure you are drinking plenty of fluids and try eating small amounts, more frequently rather than eating large meals.
- **Heartburn & indigestion** are caused by hormonal changes and, in the later stages of pregnancy, by your baby pushing against your stomach. Eating little and often can help, as well as avoiding eating too close to bedtime and cutting down on spicy or rich foods. Over-the-counter heartburn medication

is safe to use through pregnancy.
- **Bloating & constipation** are often caused by hormonal changes. Drink plenty of water, eat foods high in fibre, and try to keep some gentle exercise up to avoid too much discomfort.
- **Piles** can be common in pregnancy due to hormonal changes and can also be caused by constipation. They cause itching, soreness or swelling around your anus and occasional bleeding after you go to the toilet. Using the methods to avoid constipation (see above) and avoiding straining on the toilet can help. Holding a cold cloth over the area, or using moist toilet paper can ease discomfort.
- **Sensitive & swollen breasts** are again caused by hormonal changes as your body prepares for breastfeeding.
- **Leaking nipples** are common in the final weeks of pregnancy but can also occur months before your due date. As your body prepares for birth your breast tissue produces colostrum – a creamy, early milk – and this may leak out of your nipples before the baby is even born. Absorbent pads are available from pharmacies if required, or you could use good old-fashioned tissue inside your bra.
- **Thrush** (see page 71) can be caused by the changing bacteria balance of your vagina during pregnancy. Over-the-counter treatments are available but you

should consult your doctor or midwife before using these while you are pregnant.

- **Discharge** might increase in volume during pregnancy. Follow the advice on page 70 to determine if the colour of your discharge signals a problem.
- **Bleeding** during pregnancy can occur. It isn't always a problem, but you should always consult your doctor of midwife as it can be a sign of miscarriage (see page 115).

## Other symptoms

- **Fatigue** is particularly noticeable in the first trimester, and many women are shocked by just how exhausted they feel. Unfortunately there is no solution to this other than to get as much rest as possible. Towards the later weeks of pregnancy you might find it difficult to sleep because your baby bump prevents you lying comfortably for long. You should try to sleep on your side in the last few months of pregnancy and may find using additional pillows under your bump as support can help you to be more comfortable.
- **Increased body temperature** is caused, again, by hormonal changes and an increased blood supply to the skin. Try to wear loose, comfortable clothing in natural fibres if possible.
- **Back pain** is caused in the early stage of pregnancy by your ligaments becoming softer and stretchier. Do not hesitate to speak to your doctor if it becomes extremely uncomfortable. Occasionally, back pain in your second or third trimesters could signify early labour, so consult your doctor or midwife if you are concerned.
- **Headaches** are another early pregnancy symptom that usually gets better as your pregnancy continues. Paracetamol is safe to take in pregnancy but consult your doctor if the headaches are severe, or if they are accompanied by signs of pre-eclampsia (see Hypertension, opposite).

- **Teeth and gums** are susceptible to plaque during pregnancy if you do not follow good oral hygiene. For this reason, in the UK, NHS dental care is free to expectant mothers during pregnancy and in the first year of their baby's life. If you are suffering with vomiting (see page 117) then try to rinse your mouth with water after you have vomited to reduce acid attacking your teeth.
- **Taste and smell** can change during your pregnancy with some women experiencing an unpleasant metallic or bitter taste throughout their pregnancy, or experiencing either a loss of smell, reduced smell or noticing a persistent strong smell. (I went through this, smelling petrol and coffee wherever I went, throughout my pregnancies.)
- **Nosebleeds, a blocked nose and nasal ulcers** are other unfortunate side effects of pregnancy, caused by those hormonal changes again!
- **Pelvic pain** can be felt across the front and back of your pelvis, as well as over your perineum during pregnancy. The pain can be lessened and managed by introducing specialist exercises to strengthen the area or using a pelvic support belt. Consult your doctor or midwife for a referral to a physiotherapist.
- **Stretch marks** are very common in pregnancy and caused by stretching of the skin as your bump grows, along with hormonal changes that make skin more susceptible to stretch marks. They look like pink, red, purple or brown streaks (depending on your skin colour) and may feel itchy. Those susceptible to keloid scars may find they have more pronounced stretch marks. Although they may fade after the baby is born, they are unlikely

> Pregnancy can feel like a complete mess of unwanted side effects, but remember it doesn't last forever!

to disappear completely. There's little evidence that beauty creams can prevent stretch marks, but keeping the skin moisturized might help ease any discomfort.

- **Swollen ankles, fingers and feet** are caused by your body holding more water than usual when you are pregnant, and the extra water gathers on the lower parts of your body if you have been standing for long periods. Try to rest with your feet up wherever possible and keep up regular, gentle exercise. Gradual swelling is normal and not harmful but a sudden increase is sometimes a sign of pre-eclampsia (see Hypertension, opposite).
- **Weight gain** is caused not only by your growing baby and placenta but also by fat stores laid down to prepare your body for breastfeeding. Weight gain varies dramatically between women but most fall within the 10–12.5kg range. Try to stick to a healthy diet and gentle exercise during pregnancy. If you are worried about weight gain, do not embark on a weight-loss diet without consulting your doctor.

## Pregnancy complications

Some conditions brought on by pregnancy will require more medical attention, so alert your doctor or midwife if you experience the following:

- **Severe vomiting**, also known as hyperemesis gravidarum, is defined as vomitting many times a day and being unable to keep food and drink down. This poses a risk that you will become dehydrated and may require hospital treatment.
- **Deep vein thrombosis (DVT)** is the occurrence of a blood clot in one of the veins deep in your body and can have serious consequences. Your risk of DVT is slightly increased by pregnancy and you will be more at risk if you have an existing condition that makes clots more likely, are over 35 years old, have a family history of blood clots, smoke or are obese.
- **Gestational diabetes** is when your body cannot produce enough insulin during pregnancy and will usually be detected at a routine antenatal blood sugar screening. Your pregnancy will be closely managed and you will be given advice on controlling your blood sugar levels. It will usually go away after you have given birth.
- **Hypertension, or high blood pressure,** can be detected during routine antenatal blood pressure checks and you will be advised on how to manage it. If you have hypertension during pregnancy you are also at greater risk of pre-eclampsia, a condition in the placenta in later pregnancy, that needs to be closely monitored by your doctor.
- **Intrahepatic cholestasis** of pregnancy is a liver condition in which bile from the liver builds up in your body. Its main symptom is itching without a rash (although harmless itching is also common in pregnancy, see Stretch marks, opposite) and you'll be offered regular liver function tests, as it can potentially have serious consequences for your baby.

# Antenatal mental health

It's not unusual for women to struggle with their mental health during this pivotal time in their lives. Indeed, some may develop emotional and psychological issues for the first time during the perinatal phase, perhaps experiencing feelings they've never had before. Not only can your mood and behaviour be affected by the fluctuation of your hormones, you may naturally find yourself becoming very anxious about your unborn baby, for instance, or worrying about your future parenting skills. If these feelings become overwhelming, please don't suffer in silence; instead, speak with a healthcare professional who will assess your symptoms and signpost you to the relevant resources. You might be referred for some talking therapy, or you may be advised to join a local antenatal group where you get together with other mums-to-be.

I'm a huge advocate of self-care, too. Pregnancy can be tough, both physically and emotionally, and you shouldn't feel guilty about giving yourself some serious tender loving care.

If you already suffer with any underlying mental health conditions – such as psychosis or bipolar disorder – you should always flag these up with your doctor or midwife, who'll ensure you receive the appropriate support and monitoring with input from the obstetrics and gynaecology department.

Also, please be aware that if you're on anti-depressants and become pregnant, or are looking to conceive, there is no need to stop your medication. It is now thought that most women are safe to continue their SSRI anti-depressants throughout their pregnancy. Talk things through with your doctor, who may suggest a referral to an obstetrics and gynaecology consultant with a specialism in maternal mental health, and/or the setting up of a joint care arrangement with your psychiatrist. In addition, there are some great charities out there that offer lots of support and guidance for potential parents to care for their mental health (see Resources from page 241 for more information).

## Pregnancy TLC

Write down your thoughts in a mood diary (this can help to process your feelings).

Have a nice catch-up with a good friend, colleague or neighbour over a cup of coffee.

Give yourself half an hour to put your feet up and watch television, read a book, listen to a podcast or anything that gives you a bit of 'me time'.

# Pregnancy in Black, Asian & ethnic minority communities

I can't cover the subject of pregnancy without touching on a topic that continues to shock and sadden me. Statistics from the MBRRACE-UK group (Mothers and babies: Reducing risk through audits and confidential enquiries across the UK) show that Black women are *four* times more likely to die in pregnancy and childbirth than white women. Mixed ethnicity and Asian women are *twice* as likely to suffer this fate. And elsewhere there's a similar picture: the World Health Organization recognizes that Black and Asian women have poorer outcomes in pregnancy and post-natal care.

There can be no doubt about it: these women have been failed by the healthcare system. For decades, issues around perinatal pain (pain in pregnancy) have not been taken as seriously in Black and ethnic minority women, and birth complications haven't been picked up soon enough. This issue has been overlooked and neglected for far too long, but I'm encouraged that work is now being done to address this inequality at an institutional level, via the Department of Health and Social Care's Women's Health Strategy and the Royal College of Obstetricians and Gynaecologist's *Better for Women* report. An all–party Parliamentary group on Black maternal health has been established and, every September, Black Maternal Health Week takes place aimed at raising awareness and tackling institutionalized racism in the healthcare system.

The fundamental point is that the colour of a woman's skin should *not* impact upon her pregnancy and childbirth experience. If you believe you are not receiving the healthcare you deserve, and are not being listened to or treated with respect, you *must* flag up your concerns and make a complaint (see Resources from page 241 for organizations offering help and support). Sadly, while these inequalities persist, if you are from an ethnic minority, it becomes even more important that you are aware of your health and monitor any changes yourself (see pages 16–17 and 21–3 for advice on self examination).

**Black women in the UK are**

# 4 times

**more likely to die in pregnancy and childbirth than white women**

# Childbirth

The excitement builds as you near the end of your pregnancy, and you will have your midwife or doctor to guide you through the birth itself.

As you approach the later stages of pregnancy, you may want to write a birth plan. A birth plan outlines your ideal birth but it may need to be adjusted as the actual situation unfolds.

A birth plan may include subjects like:

- Pain relief during labour.
- Delivery positions.
- Assisted delivery preferences (forceps or a ventouse suction cup, if required during the birth).
- Location, including home, birth centre or hospital, and other preferences, such as water births.
- Timeline for holding the baby.
- Having your partner cut the umbilical cord.

You also need to decide who will be present at the birth. Some couples employ the services of a doula, a layperson who is trained as a labour companion. Doulas aren't medical professionals; their primary role is to offer emotional and physical support during labour. Doulas can be involved throughout an entire pregnancy or just for labour and delivery. They can also offer support and advice after the birth (post-partum). Talk with your partner and decide who you want to have attending the birth. Some couples feel that this is a private time and prefer not to have others present.

## Breech & transverse babies

Your baby's position inside the uterus will be checked at your pregnancy appointments. Most babies naturally turn into a head-down position towards the end of pregnancy but sometimes they will still be feet-down (breech) or lying sideways (transverse) beyond 36 weeks of pregnancy. If this is the case then your healthcare provider will discuss your options, which can include an external cephalic version, a process in which a healthcare professional will try to reposition the baby by applying pressure on your abdomen. This successfully repositions around half of breech babies but, if the baby cannot be repositioned into a head-down position, then your doctor will discuss your childbirth options, including viability of a vaginal birth or the option of a Caesarean section delivery.

## The process of childbirth

Of course every labour and birth is different, but these are the stages you will go through on your journey to parenthood.

### Amniotic sac rupture

During pregnancy, your baby sits in a fluid-filled membrane called the amniotic sac. This sac will rupture, usually before you go into labour or at the start of labour, and is commonly referred to as your 'waters breaking'. It can either feel like a gentle trickle or a sudden gush of fluid, and the fluid should be clear and odourless. When your waters break, contact the labour ward, midwife, obstetrician or other obstetric care provider and follow their guidance. Occasionally, the amniotic sac can stay intact throughout labour and the baby delivered inside the sac. Your midwife or doctor may advise that your waters are broken manually (referred to as 'artificial rupture of membranes') as the rupture of the amniotic sac can release hormones that are thought to help with labour.

### Contractions

For the baby to move through the cervix your uterine muscles will repeatedly tighten and release in a motion known as contractions. They can feel like strong period cramps or a tight internal pressure that begins in your back and moves towards the front. Contractions are likely to occur throughout labour and come closer together as your approach active labour (although their frequency can ebb and flow). A minute-long contraction, repeating itself at least five minutes apart, for an hour, is generally seen as a reliable indication that you are in active labour.

Many pregnant women will also experience contractions intermittently in their second or third trimesters, when they are not in labour. These are referred to as Braxton-Hicks contractions and mean that contractions aren't always a reliable indicator of labour.

### Stage 1: Dilation of the cervix

This first stage of active labour (and childbirth) is considered to be when your cervix has dilated 4cm or more. The cervix is a tubular structure approximately 3–4cm in length with a passage that connects the uterine cavity to the vagina. Its purpose is to keep the uterus closed through pregnancy, and then, when labour begins, it will dilate (open up) to allow the baby to be born. In the final weeks of your pregnancy, hormonal changes will cause your cervical tissue to soften and get thinner, which enables it to open more easily during labour. The cervical canal will continue opening up until it has reached 10cm in diameter and the baby is able to pass into the birth canal.

### Stage 2: The birth

Once your cervix is fully dilated to 10cm, the baby will pass through the birth canal. At this point, the skin and muscles around your vagina, labia and perineum will stretch, and you may feel a burning sensation (sometimes referred to as 'the ring of fire') when they reach their maximum stretching capacity.

Your skin and muscles may tear to allow the baby through, they may be able to stretch sufficiently on their own, or your doctor or midwife may decide to perform an episiotomy by making a small cut to the vagina to enlarge the opening. Tears and cuts can be common, particularly in a first birth, and will usually be repaired with dissolvable stitches after the placenta has been delivered.

The downwards pressure of the baby passing through your birth canal will ease as their head emerges from the vagina. The baby might need a bit of help from your midwife or doctor to clear the amniotic fluid from its lungs or its first cries might naturally clear them.

Usually, the baby's shoulders will be delivered in the next push or contraction and the midwife or doctor may rotate the baby's head slightly to make the passage of the shoulders a little easier. Once the shoulders have passed out of the vagina, the feet will easily slip out and you have delivered your baby!

### Stage 3: Delivery of the placenta

The placenta and the amniotic sac that supported and protected the baby during pregnancy will still be in the uterus after the delivery. These need to be delivered, which can happen straight away or may take a little time. Your midwife or doctor can help speed along delivery of the placenta by massaging your abdomen or offering an injection of syntometrine or syntocinon medication to stimulate its release. Delivering the placenta can cause further feelings of pressure in your uterus (although not as strong as the pressure during the birth), and you may need to push to move it through the birth canal. Your midwife or doctor will then check to ensure that all of the placenta has been safely delivered.

After delivery of the placenta, you may have an examination to determine if stitches are needed to help heal any cuts or tears from labour. Smaller cuts and tears will often heal of their own accord but the doctor may repair larger ones with stitches, that will dissolve as the body heals.

## Stage 1: Dilation of the cervix

The cervix dilates to allow your baby to pass through. Once the cervix has dilated 4cm you are considered to be in active labour and it will continue dilating up to 10cm when your baby can pass through.

**1** Before active labour, the undilated cervix is closed to safely hold your baby inside the uterus.

**2** A fully dilated cervix is 10cm or more in diameter, large enough to allow the baby to pass through ready for Stage 2, the birth.

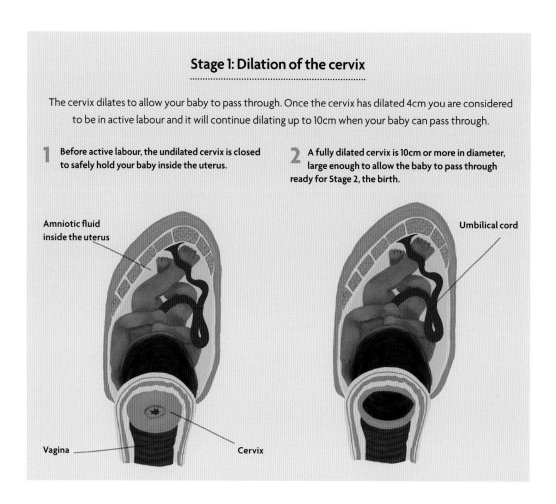

Amniotic fluid inside the uterus

Umbilical cord

Vagina

Cervix

## Stage 2: The birth

Once the cervix is fully dilated, your contractions will push the baby through the vaginal canal to be born. This stage of labour, often called the 'pushing stage', can be very hard work and you may feel an overwhelming urge to push to aid the baby on its journey.

**1** Presentation of the head as the baby passes through the vagina (birth canal) and the head emerges from the vulva.

**2** Rotation and delivery of anterior shoulder will usually occur in the next contraction after the head has emerged.

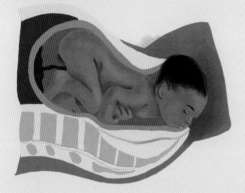

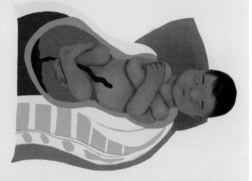

**3** Once one shoulder has emerged the baby's position will move slightly to enable the other shoulder to be released.

**4** The rest of the body will swiftly follow, with the umbilical cord remaining attached to the baby.

Placenta

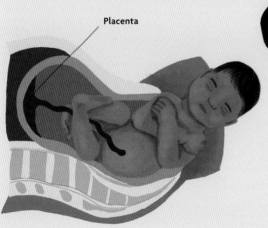

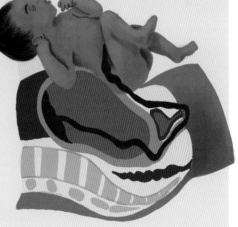

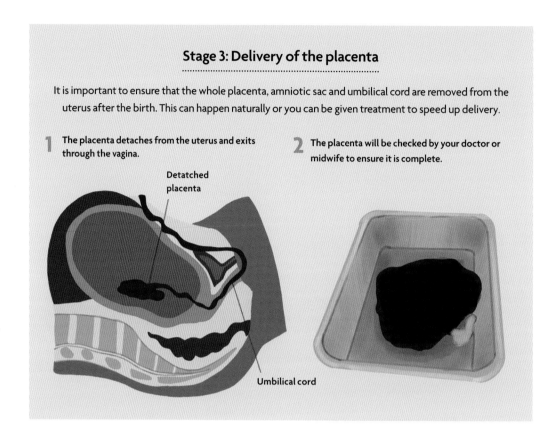

## Stage 3: Delivery of the placenta

It is important to ensure that the whole placenta, amniotic sac and umbilical cord are removed from the uterus after the birth. This can happen naturally or you can be given treatment to speed up delivery.

**1** The placenta detaches from the uterus and exits through the vagina.

**2** The placenta will be checked by your doctor or midwife to ensure it is complete.

Detatched placenta

Umbilical cord

## The moments after giving birth

The time immediately after you have given birth is very special but the experience differs significantly for different mothers. You will probably be completely exhausted or still be feeling the effects of painkilling drugs, so be gentle with yourself. Your midwife or doctor will do a check of the baby's health and, all being well, you or your partner will be given the baby to hold. Many new parents like to enjoy 'skin-to-skin' time in the first moments after the birth, where your baby's bare skin is in direct contact with your skin. This is believed to help the baby to establish breastfeeding (if that is how your choose to feed

your baby) and encourage bonding. Dads and non-birthing partners can benefit from skin-to-skin contact too so it's a wonderful time to enjoy some special moments with your new family.

The practice of placentophagy (consuming your placenta either cooked or dehydrated into capsule form) is gaining recognition as advocates believe it can help boost post-birth recovery, but there isn't any firm evidence of this.

If you gave birth in a hospital or a midwife-led unit, the length of time that you spend there after giving birth will depend on your circumstances and the baby's health, but you should be given an option to discuss how you'd like to feed the baby.

# Post-natal issues

While many post-natal conditions are addressed directly by midwives and health visitors, I will often see new mums in my surgery who have been referred to me for prescription medication to treat a variety of issues.

## Physical issues

Your body has been through a lot during pregnancy and birth, and you may experience a few of the following issues afterwards.

### Post-partum bleeding

It is common to experience some bleeding, known as lochia, for two to six weeks after birth. You should not use any internal period products (such as tampons or menstrual cups) for the first six weeks after giving birth as it could increase your chance of getting an infection. Most women will use sanitary towels, which should be changed regularly. It's also a good idea to bathe or shower daily to keep your genitals clean as they heal.

### Painful breastfeeding & mastitis

Midwives and health visitors usually work with mums to manage any breastfeeding issues in their specialized assisting clinics. However, if you are suffering with mastitis – a painful inflammation of breast tissue usually resulting from an infection – you may be referred to your family doctor to be prescribed appropriate antibiotics. The hormones released during breastfeeding can also cause vaginal atrophy (see page 168). In the first few days after birth some women also find that breastfeeding causes extreme cramps in the uterus as hormonal changes prompt the uterus to contract down to its pre-pregnancy size.

### Post-partum infections

If you are suffering with uterine, bladder or kidney infections following childbirth, you may need to be prescribed a course of antibiotics.

### Haemorrhoids & constipation

The pushing and straining of labour, and nine months of raised abdominal pressure, can cause haemorrhoids and constipation. In order to minimize these uncomfortable conditions, your doctor might advise you to follow a high-fibre diet, drink lots of water and perhaps take laxatives.

### Post-natal vaginal discharge

A thin, white, odourless vaginal discharge is normal. However, refer to page 70 for tips on when a review with your doctor may be necessary.

### Post-natal incontinence

Urge and stress incontinence is common during and after pregnancy, which is why it's always a good idea to maintain a healthy weight before you decide to have a baby. Pelvic floor exercises (see page 173) can help to tighten your muscles – and incontinence pads can make you feel more comfortable – but if you're leaking a lot of urine, don't put up with it. If it's affecting your quality of life, speak to your doctor who may be able to refer you for a scan and some urodynamic studies (tests of the lower urinary tract).

## Wellbeing after childbirth

The first year with a new baby can be a challenge. I want you to be aware of how to look after your own wellbeing and know when to ask for help.

### Post-natal depression

This mood variation can affect parents after having a baby. Symptoms include: constant sadness, difficulty bonding, lack of energy, irritability, feelings of guilt and inadequacy. New mums often experience 'baby blues' but this is short term, whereas post-natal depression is longer, more persistent and with more intrusive thoughts. It can affect both birth and non-birth parents.

### Post-partum psychosis

This affects 1 in 500 women in the UK and must be treated as a medical emergency. Symptoms are severe and usually start within the first two days, often within hours, of giving birth (although it can also develop several weeks later). Symptoms can be similar to post-natal depression but also include extreme confusion, delusions, hallucinations, paranoia and suicidal thoughts and actions, making it the leading cause of maternal death in the UK. It is under-researched, and there is a particular lack of awareness in Black and Asian communities, but the condition must be quickly assessed, treated and monitored by perinatal mental health services, as recovery is possible.

### Post-natal sex

Whenever you're ready as a couple, both in mind and body, you can start to have sex again. The emotional rollercoaster of childbirth can have a real impact on your sex life – think perineal trauma, Caesarean section scar, breastfeeding pain and sleep deprivation – so take your time, do not be pressured and seek support if needed. And be aware it is possible to become pregnant again immediately (see below).

### Post-natal contraception

If you're not breastfeeding, you can use your usual contraception (see pages 73–84). If you are breastfeeding, the IUD, barrier methods, or progesterone-only contraceptives (the POP, IUS, or contraceptive implant or injection) are recommended. It is not true that you can't get pregnant if you have just had a baby, are breastfeeding or aren't menstruating. You can!

### Post-natal menstruation

If you are not breastfeeding, periods typically return 6–12 weeks after you give birth. If you are breastfeeding, this can vary because the hormone that prompts you to make milk can prevent your body making the hormones that control menstruation so you might not bleed at all. Your periods may only resume when you stop breastfeeding completely. If your periods haven't returned within 12 months of stopping breastfeeding, see your doctor.

### Planning for another baby

Although women may be able to get pregnant just a few weeks after giving birth, this is not always safe for them or their babies. Ideally pregnancies should be spaced 18–24 months apart. This will give your body time to replenish its nutrients, heal inflammation and repair any organ damage. Getting pregnant too soon (or leaving too long between pregnancies) can result in premature birth, pre-eclampsia or placental abruption.

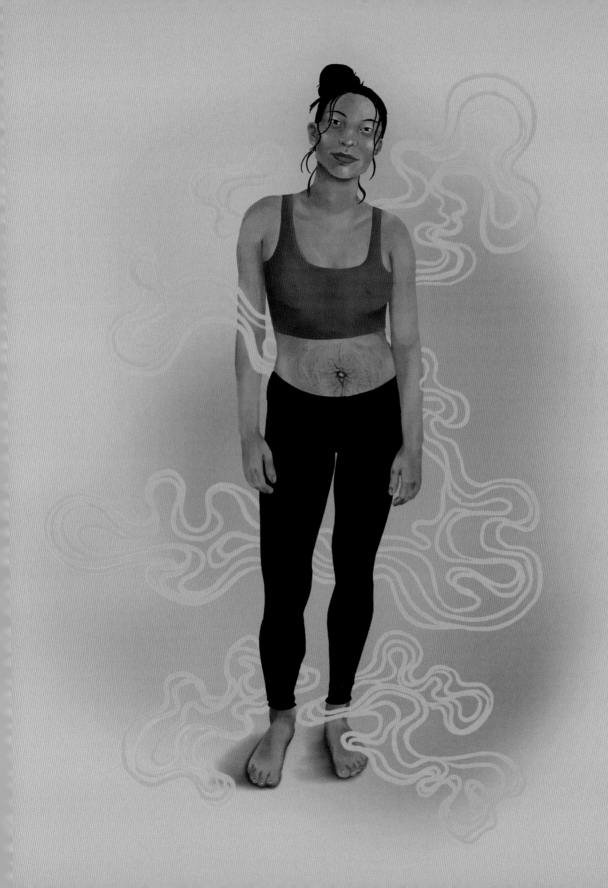

# Gynaecological areas of concern

There are a number of conditions and syndromes that can adversely affect women's health during their fertile years, but often their suffering is not investigated until they find they do not conceive as quickly as hoped. Even if you are not planning on starting a family now, or ever, I urge you to read these pages as the conditions can affect anyone, so awareness of them is vital to receiving the healthcare you deserve.

## Polycystic ovary syndrome

Polycystic ovary syndrome (PCOS) is a very common condition that affects about one in ten post-pubescent women, although over half of them don't notice any symptoms. It is thought that PCOS is associated with a hormonal imbalance; higher levels of insulin (a hormone made by the pancreas that regulates blood sugar levels) can lead to an over-production of testosterone which, in turn, affects the normal ovulation process. The development of chronic health issues, such as high cholesterol and type 2 diabetes, in later life has also been associated with having PCOS. It also seems to run in families, so you may be more at risk if your female relatives have been affected by the condition. Symptoms can often be more severe if you're obese or overweight.

Many women are given their diagnosis in their late teens and early twenties, although it can also be flagged up later when they're having problems getting pregnant. They might start monitoring their menstrual cycle and realize they have irregular periods (or no periods at all) and, as a result of haphazard or absent ovulation, they often find it difficult to conceive.

The biggest worry many women have when given a diagnosis of polycystic ovaries or polycystic ovary syndrome is that they'll have difficulty becoming pregnant. However, from my clinical experience, if the person is below the age of 35, has a healthy weight and diet and also takes clomifene citrate (clomid) or metformin (see page 107), they have a 70–80 per cent chance of becoming pregnant.

### Symptoms of PCOS

- Irregular or absent menstrual periods, which are caused by your ovaries not regularly releasing an egg.
- Excess hair (hirsutism) on your face, back, chest or buttocks, or thinning hair on the head, which is caused by excessive levels of androgen (a male hormone). This can also cause weight gain and oily skin or bad acne.
- Polycystic ovaries, which occur when your ovaries become enlarged, and multiple follicles (fluid-filled sacs) can develop. These sacs surround the egg and may prevent it from being released.

### Diagnosis of PCOS

To be diagnosed with PCOS, you need to present with at least two of the above symptoms. Despite the name of the condition, you don't actually need to have cysts in your ovaries as a qualifying factor; you could just have the irregular periods and excess androgen. Conversely and confusingly,

## Polycystic ovaries

Confusingly, you can have polycystic ovaries without having PCOS, and some women can have effects of PCOS (excessive androgen and irregular periods) without having cysts on their ovaries (see opposite for more details). The below diagram shows a polycystic ovary opposite a healthy ovary. In the healthy ovary, one follicle will mature to release an egg at ovulation each month, but in the polycystic ovary the cysts on the ovary are swollen and sore. Because there are a number of cysts, the follicles can be prevented from maturing so no egg is released and ovulation does not occur.

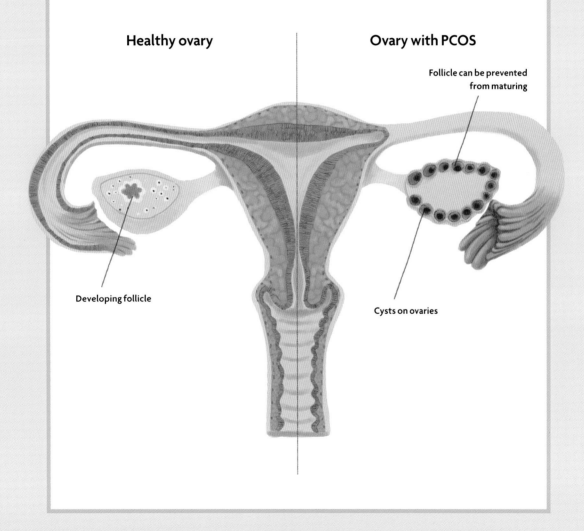

**Healthy ovary**

**Ovary with PCOS**

Follicle can be prevented from maturing

Developing follicle

Cysts on ovaries

you can also have polycystic ovaries without having the syndrome; some women may possess a large number of harmless follicles in their ovaries (up to 8mm in size), but don't present with irregular periods and/or excess androgen.

### Treatment of PCOS

There is no cure for PCOS, but it can be managed. Treatment is more often than not based around individual symptoms, for example a person with a high BMI might embark on a weight-loss programme, usually incorporating a healthy, balanced diet. Someone with insulin resistance may receive similar advice, but may also be prescribed the drug metformin, which is commonly used to treat people with type 2 diabetes.

A patient with menstrual irregularities can take the combined or progesterone-only contraceptive pill or, if they prefer, can be fitted with an IUS coil (see page 79). Excessive hair growth on the face and body can be addressed with ruby laser treatment or, alternatively, with a topical eflornithine cream or an anti-androgen medication (such as spironolactone).

An individual with severe acne can often respond well to a medication called Dianette (which also has contraceptive properties) because it has high levels of anti-androgens. However these benefits will have to be weighed up for a person with a BMI of over 30, because of the increased risk of blood clots.

Once diagnosed with PCOS, you should be monitored for early signs of health problems. This may involve the following:

- **Regular blood pressure checks** which you can do at home before discussing the readings with your doctor. Blood pressure monitors can be purchased easily, and you may find it useful to keep a diary of the readings; there's a great one to download and print from the British Hypertension Society (see Resources from page 241).
- **Diabetes checks** will be undertaken depending on your weight, lifestyle, BMI and family history. You may be entitled to an HbA1c diabetes blood test and a fasting cholesterol test every one to three years.
- **Checks for cancer of the uterus** should ideally be undertaken every three to four months to check for any thickening of the lining of the uterus and to therefore reduce the chances of uterine cancer. If you've not had a period for four months and you're not on contraceptives to stop your periods, talk to your doctor. They may be able to give you a medication such as a contraceptive to regulate your period, or might send you for an ultrasound scan to check the lining of the uterus.

### Living with PCOS

If you feel PCOS has affected your mood or has caused depression, you can either bring it up with your doctor or self-refer to your local Healthy Minds service (usually contactable via your local NHS foundation trust website) where you may benefit from talking therapy.

Women with PCOS tend to reach menopause about two years later than the average, but symptoms of PCOS do not disappear with menopause. Testosterone levels will decrease in post-menopause but from a higher point than in women without PCOS. Small studies have found that testosterone levels in post-menopausal women are roughly equal, in those with and without PCOS, about 20 years after menopause.

## Adenomyosis

Adenomyosis is a little-known (and much misdiagnosed) condition that sees the inner lining of the uterus (endometrium) breaking into the muscle wall of the uterus (myometrium), causing it to thicken and stiffen.

Like endometriosis (see page 136), this not an infection, it's not contagious, and it's a benign (not cancerous) condition. Nobody is quite sure why it occurs, but it's likely that most sufferers will have a genetic predisposition to it. About one-third of women with adenomyosis experience few or no symptoms whatsoever; it's often picked up by chance during an ultrasound scan checking for another condition.

Adenomyosis may be less recognizable than endometriosis, but it still affects a significant number of people; it's thought that one in ten women have it, more commonly women in their forties and fifties who have had children. That said, in my clinical practice I've seen many patients in their twenties and thirties who present to me with pelvic pain and heavy periods, who are eventually diagnosed with adenomyosis. Very sadly, some have suffered miscarriages. Maintaining a pregnancy can be more difficult if the uterus lining is stiffened and the uterus is prevented from expanding, so anyone with adenomyosis may be at higher risk of losing their baby or having a premature birth. They may require close monitoring from a specialist consultant.

Research on this is scant, but it's thought that adenomyosis is unlikely to hinder conception and fertility. Unlike endometriosis, it doesn't usually cause scarring to the fallopian tubes and ovaries, which can hinder eggs from travelling towards sperm for fertilization.

### Symptoms of adenomyosis

- Severe menstrual cramps.
- Heavy or painful periods and irregular periods.
- Irregular periods.
- Pelvic pain.
- Pressure or discomfort in the lower abdomen.
- Bloating before your period.
- Pain during or after sex.
- Severe anaemia (due to heavy periods).

### Diagnosis of adenomyosis

It can take many years to diagnose adenomyosis. Being such an obscure and unrecognized condition, it often gets missed or misdiagnosed as severe period pain (dysmenorrhea) or uterine fibroids (see page 141) and, in some cases, is confused with endometriosis. A transvaginal ultrasound scan of the pelvis can assist with the diagnosis, but this tends to happen only when the condition is in its advanced stages, when the uterine walls have become extremely thickened, and by which time the patient may have suffered horrendously for years. Other than this, the condition is detected by a laparoscopy (see page 140) or an MRI scan.

### Treatment of adenomyosis

As with endometriosis, there is no cure for adenomyosis, but we as family doctors can help to manage a patient's pain and discomfort. For those at the milder end of the pain spectrum, a combination of painkillers and hormonal contraceptives can help to keep symptoms at bay, as can the addition of some lifestyle changes (diet, exercise, and so on).

I'll usually discuss the following treatment pathways with my adenomyosis patients in order

## Effects of adenomyosis

The endometrium is the lining of the uterus that thickens and breaks away during a menstrual cycle; it is encased in a muscle wall called the myometrium. Adenomyosis is a condition that sees the endometrium lining breaking into and embedding itself into the myometrium. This causes the myometrium to thicken and can result in feelings of pain, pressure and bloating, severe menstrual cramps, heavy and irregular periods, anaemia or pain during sex.

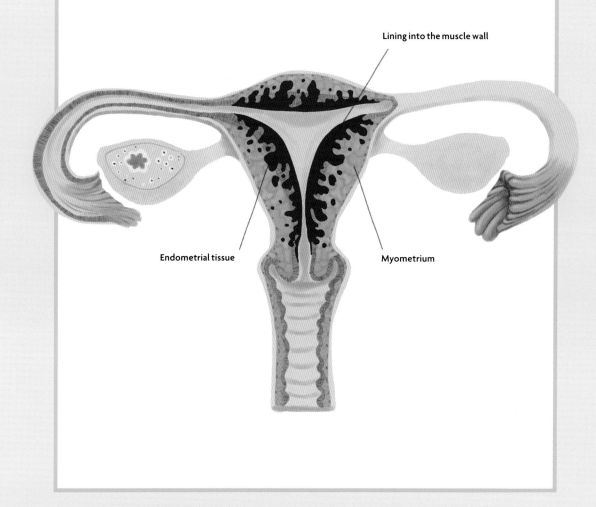

Lining into the muscle wall

Endometrial tissue

Myometrium

to ascertain what best suits their needs (most of the options are similar to those offered for endometriosis). As always with women's health, there's rarely a one-size-fits-all solution.

- **Pain relief** (paracetamol and/or ibuprofen, if the latter can be tolerated).
- **Hormone regulation treatment** (for example, oral contraceptive pill, implant, injection or IUS coil).
- **Mefenamic acid**, which can help with pain and bleeding, if tolerated.
- **Tranexamic acid**, a medication prescribed for heavy periods that can reduce pain and bleeding.
- **Ablation**, a surgical procedure that involves burning away a layer on the inside of the uterus, which can reduce or eliminate heavy bleeding.
- **Hysterectomy**, the surgical removal of the uterus, can be an option for severe cases of adenomyosis.

Hysterectomy is the only sure-fire way of permanently ridding yourself of severe adenomyosis. This is often a viable treatment for older women, but is not always preferable for young, fertile women who aim to get pregnant one day. Sadly, family doctors such as myself often find themselves having very frank conversations with patients who are desperate to rid themselves of the pain and suffering associated with adenomyosis (and endometriosis), but who are still keen to have babies; it's a heart-rending dilemma to face. There is a little piece of light at the end of the tunnel, though; adenomyosis symptoms tend to improve as women in their forties and fifties transition into the menopause.

## Living with adenomyosis

The painful symptoms associated with adenomyosis, especially if it left untreated, can detrimentally affect your physical and emotional wellbeing. If the heavy periods and pelvic pain aren't bad enough to contend with, there's also a debilitating and uncomfortable condition called 'adenomyosis belly'. This is caused when the uterine walls grow and thicken, putting pressure on surrounding organs like the bladder and intestine. This in turn leads to a bloated, protruding abdomen which, for obvious reasons, can have a terrible effect on someone's self-confidence. I know a lot of women who've been told by their doctors that they've got a bad case of IBS (irritable bowel syndrome), or have just put on weight, but who've then gone on to get a diagnosis of adenomyosis. This is the reason why we desperately need to increase research and awareness!

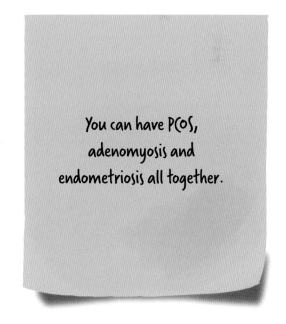

You can have PCOS, adenomyosis and endometriosis all together.

## Endometriosis

Endometriosis is a condition that occurs when microscopic cells similar to those found in the lining of the uterus – known as the endometrium – are distributed around the pelvis and abdomen. During a woman's menstrual cycle, these cells behave in the same way as those in the uterus by building up and breaking down. However, unlike the cells of the uterus – which are evacuated from the body as a period – this tissue has no way of escaping; it instead grows outside the uterus, remaining attached to different areas of the body that may include:

- The ovaries and the fallopian tubes.
- The outer side of the uterus.
- The lining of the inside of the abdomen.
- The bowel or bladder.

These growths can cause severe pain and inflammation, and can sometimes lead to scarring (also known as fibrous adhesions).

In the UK, it is estimated that one in ten women are living with endometriosis. It's a condition that can affect you from your teenage years to your midlife years. Most sufferers are diagnosed between the ages of 25 and 40 – although, for many, the impact can have lasting repercussions. It is thought that the condition may be passed through the genes, so if your mum or an aunt has the condition, you may well be more susceptible. Having dealt with numerous cases of endometriosis in my surgery, I know just how distressing and debilitating it can be.

### Symptoms of endometriosis

- Painful or heavy periods (with or without clots).
- Pain during or after sex (particularly if penetration is deep).
- Pain during ovulation.
- Painful bowel movements.
- Sharp or burning pain during or following a bowel movement, that's especially prevalent during your period.
- Pain when passing urine.
- Leg pain and cramps.
- Back pain.
- Bowel and bladder pain, in some cases due to endometrial adhesions.
- Diarrhoea, constipation and bloating.
- Fatigue and lack of energy.
- Infertility.
- Depression.

### Diagnosis of endometriosis

On average, it takes about seven years – yes, you read that correctly, *seven years* – for a woman to receive a confirmed endometriosis diagnosis. This is often the case because its signs and symptoms can be mistaken for other conditions like heavy periods (see page 65). The diagnostic process will start with your doctor who, after obtaining a full medical history from you, may carry out an internal pelvic examination or recommend an ultrasound scan to detect ovarian cysts or scar tissue that may have been caused by endometriosis. It's not always straightforward, however, because an ultrasound scan can be reported as normal and yet the patient can have endometriosis. Some patients are referred to a gynaecologist for a laparoscopy, a minor operation performed under general anaesthetic in which a camera is inserted into the pelvis. Endometriosis can only be confirmed with this surgical examination; the consultant will take a biopsy that will be examined very carefully to look for signs of

# Effects of endometriosis

The endometrium is the lining of the uterus that thickens and breaks away during a menstrual cycle. Endometriosis refers to a condition in which tiny cells, similar to those of the endometrial lining, break away from their usual position and embed themselves in other areas of the abdomen. The diagram below shows some of the places where these cells can situate themselves.

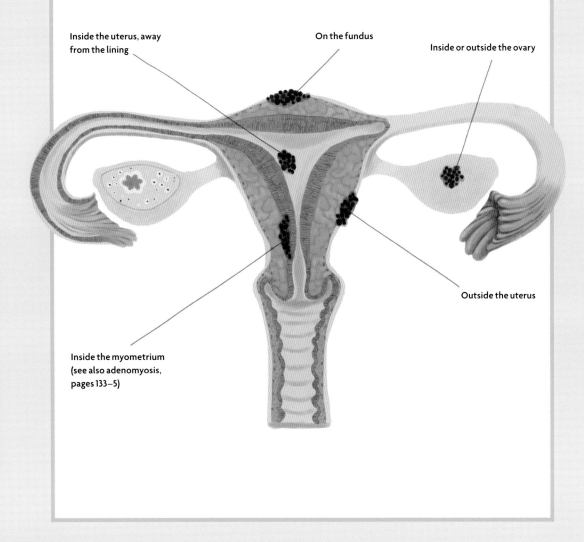

Inside the uterus, away from the lining

On the fundus

Inside or outside the ovary

Outside the uterus

Inside the myometrium (see also adenomyosis, pages 133–5)

## Endometriosis in the bladder & bowel

Endometriosis is not exclusive to the reproductive system and the condition can cause cells similar to those in the endometrial lining to cluster on the bladder or bowel. In rare cases endometriosis can also spread as far as the heart and lungs (not pictured here). The diagram below shows some of the places where these cells can situate themselves.

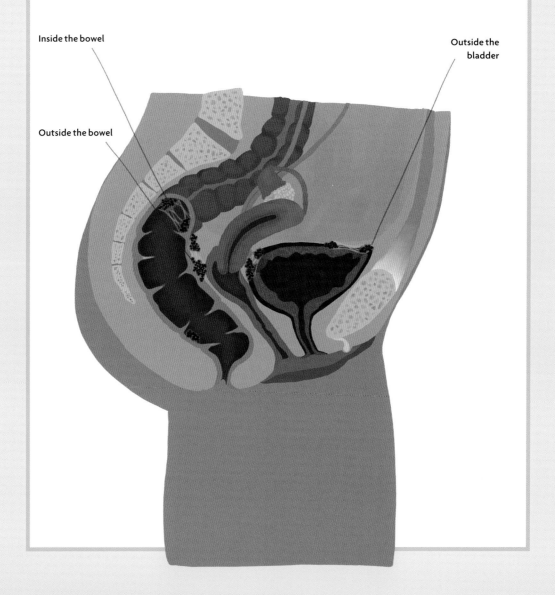

Inside the bowel

Outside the bladder

Outside the bowel

the condition. This is currently the gold-standard method of diagnosing endometriosis.

Infuriatingly, far too many women are suffering needlessly with endometriosis because they haven't been taken seriously enough by a clinician. Do not let anyone normalize or trivialize your pain and, ideally, back up your case and empower yourself with personal data from a tracker app (or a diary) on which you record your symptoms each month. Monitoring how painful or heavy your periods are will make it easier for you and your doctor to see if there are any patterns emerging. If you still feel you're not being listened to, you have the right to change your doctor, preferably to one with a special interest in women's health.

### Treating endometriosis

Since there is no cure for endometriosis, treatment isn't straightforward. Some women opt for pain management to ease the symptoms and improve their quality of life, whereas others undergo surgery to prevent the condition from returning. Another way to prevent symptoms of endometriosis is to get pregnant which obviously may not always be possible or feasible for some women.

All of the following treatment options need to be discussed with your doctor, who will outline the various risks and benefits:

- **Pain relief** (paracetamol and/or ibuprofen, if the latter can be tolerated).
- **Hormone treatment** to slow the growth of the endometrial tissue (oral contraceptive pill, implant, injection or IUS coil).
- **Tranexamic acid**, a medication prescribed for heavy periods that can reduce pain and bleeding.

- **Ablation**, a surgical procedure that involves burning away a layer on the inside of the uterus, which can reduce or eliminate heavy bleeding.
- **Laparoscopic (keyhole) surgery** (see pages 107 and 140) for fertility improvement.
- **Hysterectomy** to prevent the disease.

My hope is that, in the future, with more research, endometriosis will be diagnosed easily and rapidly through the detection of bio markers – in other words, molecules found in blood, fluids or tissue that can flag up certain diseases or conditions. Endometriosis UK has a fabulous website for those needing more information (see Resources from page 241).

### Living with endometriosis

The emotional and physical impact of endometriosis can be significant. The chronic pain can badly affect wellbeing, with work life, family life and social life often suffering as a consequence. Any difficulty you may have becoming pregnant – which may or may not be linked to the condition – will only pile on the pressure and trauma.

The lack of research means that, as things stand, we're unclear as to whether endometriosis directly causes infertility, although some do believe it may be associated with fertility problems, perhaps stemming from damage and scarring to reproductive organs. That being said, you shouldn't fear the worst if you receive an endometriosis diagnosis; even those with severe cases can go on to have a healthy baby.

# Laparoscopic surgery for endometriosis

Laparoscopic (keyhole) surgery can be used to treat endometriosis. Under a general anaesthetic, a small incision is made into your abdomen and carbon dioxide gas is passed into the abdomen to inflate the area. The surgeon will then insert a laparoscope (a small telescope) through the incision in order to view the patches of endometriosis. These patches are then either surgically removed through a second incision or destroyed with electrosurgical heat treatment.

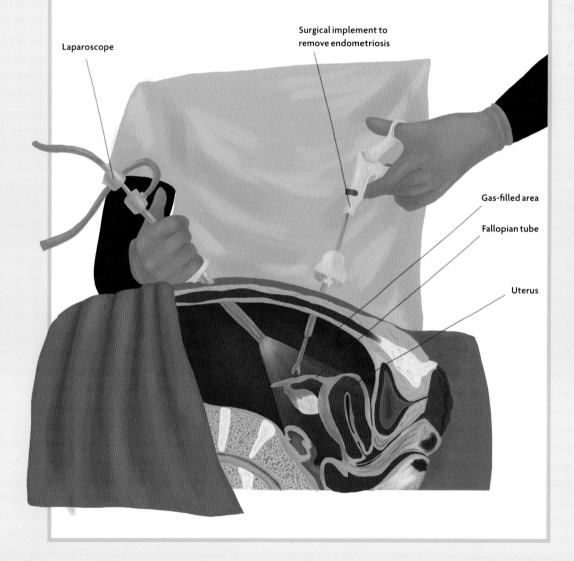

Laparoscope

Surgical implement to remove endometriosis

Gas-filled area

Fallopian tube

Uterus

## Uterine fibroids

Uterine fibroids (leiomyomas) are non-cancerous growths of the uterus. They're not associated with an increased risk of uterine cancer and do not usually develop into tumours. Fibroids vary hugely in size, from tiny growths that are invisible to the human eye, to really large masses that can be seen clearly on an ultrasound or MRI scan. A woman can develop a single fibroid or multiple fibroids; in extreme cases, a number of growths can expand into the uterus, adding weight to the abdomen and making you feel bloated, almost like you're pregnant.

Uterine fibroids are extremely common, so much so that one in three women will get them in their lifetime. We don't really know why they develop but we think it's linked to the hormone oestrogen, fluctuations of which can thicken the lining of the uterus, so they are more likely to occur during your fertile years when hormonal imbalances, variations or swings, especially of oestrogen, can be at their highest. Women who've had children have a lower risk of developing the condition, and the risk decreases with the more children you have. Fibroids tend to shrink as the menopause approaches and oestrogen levels decline. Those with Mediterranean or Afro-Caribbean heritage are said to be more susceptible to fibroids, as are obese or overweight women (excess weight causes an increased level of oestrogen in the body).

### Symptoms of uterine fibroids

- Heavy periods.
- Painful periods.
- Stomach pain.
- Lower back pain.
- Bloating.
- Frequent need to urinate (as the mass presses on the bladder).
- Constipation.
- Pain or discomfort during sex.

Many people, however, don't even realize they have fibroids and often the growths will be shed with their uterine lining during menstruation.

In rarer cases, fibroids can hamper your chances of conceiving a baby, particularly if the fibroid is situated in the lining of the uterus and is somehow affecting implantation. The pregnancy itself can be affected by fibroids – they can hinder the growth of the baby – and, in some instances, they can cause infertility. Depending on their size and whereabouts, fibroids can act as 'foreign bodies', thus causing an obstruction between the egg and sperm or preventing implantation.

By age 35, **60% of Black women** are thought to have uterine fibroids, compared to 6% of white women

## Possible sites & types of uterine fibroids

Uterine fibroids are non-cancerous growths of the uterus and can vary hugely in size. There are several types of fibroid depending on their placement within the reproductive system: subserosal fibroids develop outside the wall of the uterus and grow into the pelvis; submucosal fibroids develop in the layer of muscle that lies beneath the lining of the uterus and can then push the walls of the uterus inwards; intramural fibroids develop inside the muscle walls of the uterus; intracavitary fibroids develop inside the cavity of the uterus; and pedunculated fibroids grow inside or outside the uterus, attached by a thin stalk of tissue.

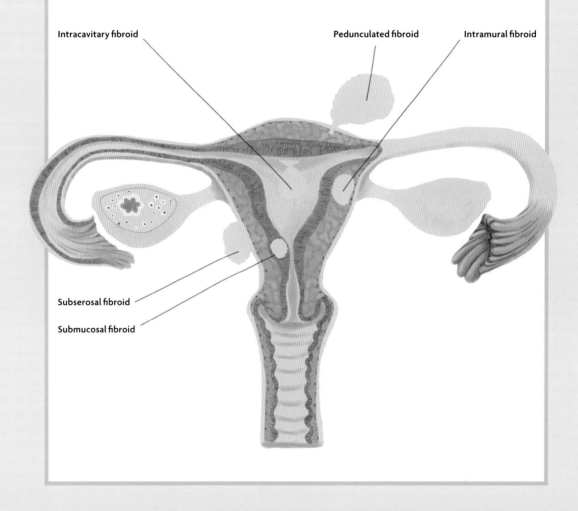

Intracavitary fibroid

Pedunculated fibroid

Intramural fibroid

Subserosal fibroid

Submucosal fibroid

## Bi-manual examination for fibroids

Uterine fibroids are diagnosed with a bi-manual examination. During the examination the doctor will insert the fingers of one hand into the vaginal canal, place the other hand on the outside of the abdomen and palpate their hands in order to feel for fibroids inside or around the uterus.

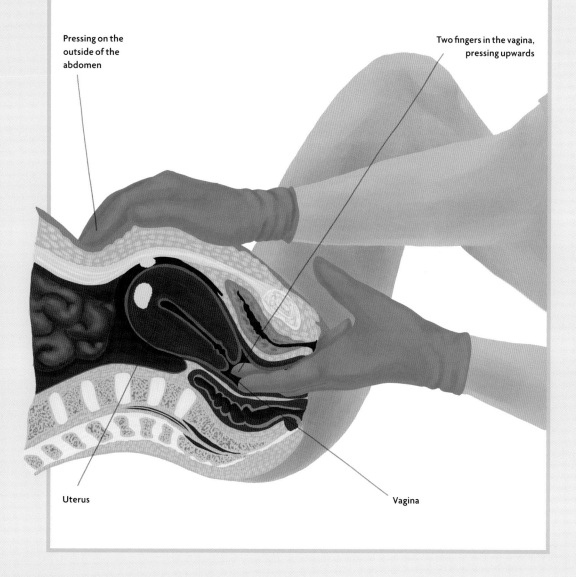

Pressing on the outside of the abdomen

Two fingers in the vagina, pressing upwards

Uterus

Vagina

### Diagnosis of fibroids

If any of the symptoms listed on page 141 become problematic, speak to your doctor. They'll usually perform what's known as a bi-manual examination (see page 143), which involves palpating (feeling) the uterus to check for any bulkiness or any anomalies. Sometimes, patients will be referred for an ultrasound scan for further investigation.

### Treatment of fibroids

Subsequent treatment depends on the site and severity of the fibroids. More often than not they don't need treating, since they shrink over time and are often shed with periods. Implementing lifestyle changes – like losing weight, stopping smoking and cutting down alcohol – can also help some women. The symptoms of pain and heavy bleeding can be managed by the combined oral contraceptive pill or the mini-pill (POP), or by LARCS (long-acting reversible contraceptives) such as the IUS progesterone coil, implant or injection. In more serious cases, we can try to shrink fibroids with hormone injections, or you can have minor surgery (fibroidectomy or myomectomy) to scrape away the lining of the uterus. The latter can be a suitable option if you're in your fertile years and are planning to have children.

A uterine ablation (a procedure to remove a thin layer of tissue) or a uterine fibroid embolization (when the blood supply to the fibroids is cut off) can also be performed, although the risks and benefits to your fertility would need to be weighed up by you and your clinician. In extreme cases, a hysterectomy may be an option for those women who fully understand the implications of uterus-removal surgery.

## Other issues

PCOS, adenomyosis, endometriosis and uterine fibroids are the more common (although still undiagnosed in many cases) conditions that can affect women in their fertile years, but there are a couple of more general conditions.

### Pelvic inflammatory disease

Pelvic inflammatory disease (PID) is the general term for inflammation of the upper genital tract of the female reproductive system, including the uterus, the ovaries, the fallopian tubes and other connecting tissues. PID is often caused by a bacterial infection, which in many cases stems from a sexually transmitted disease (STD) such as chlamydia or gonorrhoea (see pages 87–9).

It's possible that PID can lead to pregnancy-related complications. Occasionally the fallopian tubes can be left narrowed and scarred, which may increase the chances of an ectopic pregnancy (see page 115). Someone with untreated or persistent PID may also be more likely to experience fertility issues; that being said, many of my patients who've had PID have been able to conceive and carry a baby without significant problems.

### Early menopause

Early (or premature) menopause, which may occur for a variety of reasons, will have a significant impact on fertility and can affect your ability to have children naturally. There are more details about this on page 164.

# Vulval & vaginal pain

You may encounter pain in your vulva or vagina due to one of these conditions or as a result of FGM (see page 68). Please also be aware that skin conditions in particular are often harder to diagnose among Black and Asian women with darker skin. Be persistent with your doctor if you are concerned!

## Pelvic organ prolapse

Vaginal pain can occasionally be caused by a debilitating condition known as pelvic organ prolapse. This occurs when the uterus or the bladder slips down from its normal position and presses onto the vagina, causing a bulge.

A prolapse is not life-threatening but it can cause significant pain and discomfort, particularly in and around the vagina, making sex difficult and causing bladder leakage. While symptoms can vary in severity at different stages of your monthly cycle, or during or after exercise, sometimes they are ever-present.

Whereas pelvic organ prolapse is more likely to occur among post-menopausal women, it can also affect women in their twenties and thirties, particularly those with a high BMI (body mass index). Carrying extra weight can add pressure to the pelvic organs and can subsequently impact upon the vagina.

### Symptoms of pelvic organ prolapse

- A feeling of heaviness around the lower abdomen and genitals.
- A visible lump or bulge in the vagina.
- Vaginal dryness.
- A dragging sensation in the vagina; some women say it feels like sitting on a small ball.
- Discomfort or numbness during sex.
- Difficulty passing urine.

- Urinary tract infection (UTI) symptoms such as burning when passing urine, pain on passing urine, blood in the urine, increased frequency of passing urine, incomplete emptying, passing more urine than usual at night, lower abdominal pain, fever.
- Abdominal discomfort.
- Backache.

### Diagnosis of pelvic organ prolapse

If you're worried you have a prolapse, please get yourself checked out. Your doctor may perform an internal pelvic examination using a vaginal speculum or they'll do a bi-manual examination using both hands (see page 143). Sometimes your doctor will ask you to cough to see how pronounced the bulge is. They might also ask you to lie on your side in order to get a better view of the prolapse.

### Treatment of pelvic organ prolapse

For milder cases, treatment is primarily related to implementing lifestyle changes and, as such, can take a while to have an effect.

- **Lose weight** if you're overweight, especially if your BMI is over 30. Your doctor will encourage you to follow a healthy eating plan.
- **Avoid heavy lifting** as much as possible, although I know this just isn't practical in real life – especially if you have children. Instead I ask my patients, as part of their rehab, to ask themselves, 'Do I need to be

doing this lifting?' and to opt out if at all possible, perhaps delegating the task to someone else.

- **Follow a programme of specialized pelvic floor exercises** (see page 173), that your doctor can recommend. Pelvic floor muscle training helps to improve strength, endurance and coordination in that area (I often tell my patients to compare the pelvic floor with the foundations of a house – it provides stability and support for what is above). A programme of supervised physiotherapy is also suggested for at least 16 weeks for symptomatic women with grade 1 or 2 prolapses. Pilates can be very helpful, too, especially in the post-natal period.

- **Look after your bowel and bladder** by sitting on the toilet rather than hovering, so your muscles can relax. Try not to strain when you're having a poo; if you're struggling to empty your bowels, perform a 'double voiding', which means having an initial wee, then standing up, then sitting back down before trying to poo again. To avoid constipation, preventative measures such as drinking more water and eating more fruit and vegetables may help, as well as taking laxatives if needed. You might even consider investing in a footstool so that you can position your body in a comfortable squatting position on the toilet, to aid healthy bowel movements. No need to rush things…just take your time!

- **Try topical vaginal oestrogen** to help with vaginal muscle tone, which can be affected by prolapses.

- **Use a vaginal pessary** if your pelvic organ prolapse is severe. A vaginal pessary is a soft, removable device (usually made from silicone) which is inserted inside the vagina in order to support the prolapsed walls of the vagina or uterus. It is usually inserted by a nurse or doctor, but some patients get the knack of inserting it themselves. Various shapes and sizes, such as ring pessaries or shelf pessaries, are available to suit individual needs. Women may choose a pessary for severe prolapses if they wish to avoid surgery but, on the downside, they can sometimes make sexual intercourse uncomfortable.

Some women don't respond well to preliminary treatment, and their quality of life suffers badly as a result. A doctor may decide to refer these patients to a gynaecologist, who will decide whether surgery is feasible. Options can include a sacrospinous fixation, which is an operation performed under general anaesthetic to stitch the top of the vagina or the cervix to a pelvic ligament, providing support to the pelvic floor. Vaginal mesh, which was once used to treat pelvic organ prolapse, is now banned in the UK. The other surgical option is a vaginal hysterectomy, a procedure that is less invasive than an abdominal hysterectomy and involves the removal of the cervix and the uterus via an incision in the vagina, thus removing the downward pressure of those organs. Your doctor should discuss the implications of uterus–removal surgery with you first.

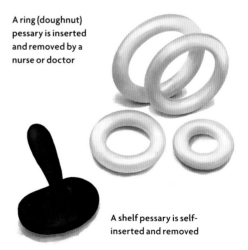

A ring (doughnut) pessary is inserted and removed by a nurse or doctor

A shelf pessary is self-inserted and removed

## Lichen sclerosus

Lichen sclerosus is a little-known, eczema-like skin condition that affects the vulva and perineum. It is not contagious.

### Symptoms of lichen sclerosus

- Itchy red or white patches on the vulva or the perineum.
- Red, sore and inflamed, or bleeding (if rubbed) patches on the vulva or perineum.

### Diagnosis of lichen sclerosus

Lichen sclerosus is usually diagnosed after examination by your doctor and discussion of your symptoms, although a biopsy may also be requested. If the patches change in size and shape, or are an enlarging lump that fails to heal, there is a small risk (around five per cent) of developing squamous cell carcinoma, a type of skin cancer. So it's imperative that you seek medical advice as soon as possible. I know no one relishes the idea of their genitalia being examined, but your health *must* outweigh any feelings of embarrassment. Your doctor will do all they can to make you feel as comfortable as possible and you can request a female doctor if you prefer.

### Treatment of lichen sclerosus

- **Wearing cotton underwear** for better air flow.
- **Applying a vaginal moisturizer** and/or emollients.
- **Applying a prescribed steroid cream** (clobetasol propionate or diflucortolone valerate).
- **Using an oil-based vaginal lubricant** or a water-based vaginal moisturizer during sexual intercourse.
- **A prescribed low-dose neuropathic painkiller**, such as amitriptyline or gabapentin.

### Effects of lichen sclerosus

Lichen sclerosus is a non-contagious, eczema-like skin condition on the vulva. It shows as itchy, sore white and/or red patches on the vulva or perineum and is more difficult to diagnose on darker skin. Below it is shown as white patches on the clitoral hood, clitoris, labia minora, perinium and rectum.

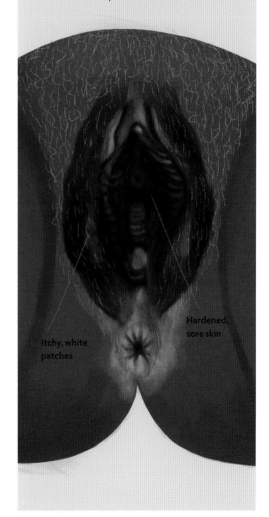

Itchy, white patches

Hardened, sore skin

## Lichen planus

Lichen planus is a condition that can affect many areas of the skin including the vulva. It is not contagious and breastfeeding women can often suffer with lichen planus–like symptoms connected to hormone fluctuation.

### Symptoms of lichen planus

- Soreness, burning and 'raw' sensation on the vulva.
- White streaks covering the vulva.
- Broken or split skin with painful red patches that can make sexual intercourse very uncomfortable.

### Diagnosis of lichen planus

Lichen planus is usually diagnosed after examination by your doctor and discussion of your symptoms, although a biopsy may also be requested.

### Treatment of lichen planus

- **Wearing cotton underwear** for better air flow.
- **Applying a vaginal moisturizer** and/or emollients.
- **Applying a prescribed steroid cream** (clobetasol propionate or diflucortolone valerate).
- **Using an oil-based vaginal lubricant** or a water-based vaginal moisturizer during sexual intercourse.
- **A prescribed low-dose neuropathic painkiller**, such as amitriptyline or gabapentin.
- **Low-dose vaginal oestrogen** (as a three-to-six-month course for breastfeeding women, or continual for perimenopausal women).

## Effects of lichen planus

Lichen planus is a non-contagious skin condition on the vulva. Below it is shown as white streaks on the labia minora and bright red, sore patches around the vulva, clitoris and vagina.

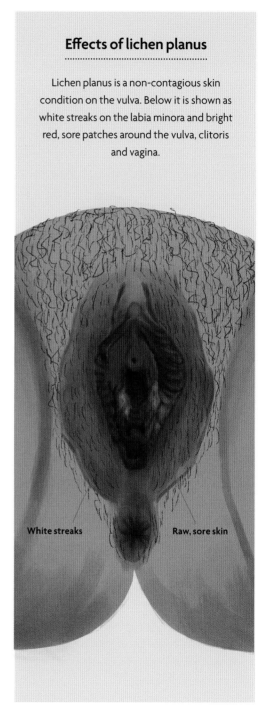

White streaks

Raw, sore skin

## Vulvodynia

This condition is characterized by pain and discomfort in and around the vulval, vaginal and groin area, and can be classified as one of two types: unprovoked or generalized vulvodynia and provoked vulvodynia. Vulvodynia can be distressing, especially if you're in a sexual relationship, and it's believed that one-quarter of women will experience it at some point in their lives.

### Symptoms of vulvodynia

- Continuous burning, stinging or soreness of the vulva or groin area (known as unprovoked vulvodynia, see pink annotations, right).
- Pain experienced at the entrance to the vagina, the vulva or the clitoris when pressure is applied (known as provoked vulvodynia, see blue annotations, right). This may occur during sex or when inserting a tampon or menstrual cup.

### Diagnosis of vulvodynia

A diagnosis of vulvodynia may be given by your doctor if all tests for infections come back negative, yet you continue to suffer with pain, burning or soreness.

### Treatment of vulvodynia

There is no specific treatment for vulvodynia. Research into the condition is shockingly limited, but any underlying vulval/vaginal conditions such as vaginal atrophy (see page 168), lichen sclerosus (see page 147) or lichen planus (see opposite) can be helped with a low dose of a medication called amitriptyline. The dose may be adjusted according to the response. The health and lifestyle tweaks for good vulval/vaginal health (see page 69) should also help to alleviate symptoms.

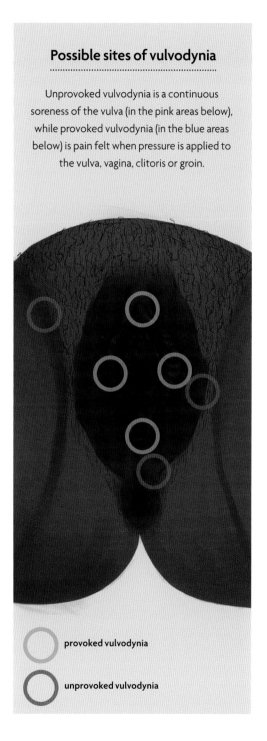

### Possible sites of vulvodynia

Unprovoked vulvodynia is a continuous soreness of the vulva (in the pink areas below), while provoked vulvodynia (in the blue areas below) is pain felt when pressure is applied to the vulva, vagina, clitoris or groin.

provoked vulvodynia

unprovoked vulvodynia

# Gynaecological cancers

There are a number of gynaecological cancers that only affect women and trans people assigned female at birth and it is important to be aware of them. Being told you have cancer is everyone's worst nightmare. According to NHS research conducted in 2022, nearly six in ten of us admit that cancer is our greatest health fear, eclipsing other illnesses such as heart disease.

Prompt diagnosis is key to combatting this dreadful disease, of course, as is increased public awareness, and regular self examination is vital (see pages 21–3). However, far too many people with warning signs and tell-tale symptoms are reluctant to seek medical help by visiting their doctor. By putting things off – and perhaps convincing themselves they're okay, and that cancer only happens to other people – thousands of individuals each week are missing out on early, life-saving intervention.

In the survey, over two-fifths of people (42 per cent) admitted to putting off an appointment by either ignoring their symptoms, waiting to see if anything changed, looking for answers online or speaking to family and friends.

**Your doctor wants to see you!**

Please do not delay phoning for an appointment if you have a persistent problem that's been playing on your mind. You may be losing weight for no apparent reason, for example, or you may be aware of a lump in your breast or a sore on your vulva. It might be nothing serious, but you're not losing anything by getting checked out by a clinician.

If something doesn't feel right to you and doesn't seem better after three weeks, please see your doctor. Keep a diary if you can to track your symptoms: keep track of your period, your eating habits, your weight, your bowel movements. And when you speak to the receptionist, have the confidence to say 'I'm bleeding between periods and I'm scared it might be cervical cancer', because your specific concerns will then be flagged up to the doctor. Being forewarned in this way will help your doctor to zone in on your symptoms and optimize that initial appointment.

As a doctor with a specialist interest in women's health, I'm particularly keen to raise awareness of the five main gynaecological cancers:

- Ovarian
- Vulval
- Vaginal
- Cervical
- Uterine

It can be very difficult to spot the warning signs associated with these cancers, especially ovarian cancer. Because of this, some women can receive a relatively late diagnosis – at stage 3 or stage 4, when the disease is severe with a poor prognosis. Tragically, many will lose their lives. Gynaecological cancer mortality rates need to be reduced, and doctors like myself are doing our utmost to encourage women to recognize the key symptoms and seek the appropriate help.

# Where gynaecological cancers can occur

There are five main gynaecological cancers. These areas are highlighted below and it is possible for cancerous cells to grow in the uterus (uterine cancer), one or both ovaries (ovarian cancer), the cervix (cervical cancer), the vagina (vaginal cancer) or the vulva (vulval cancer).

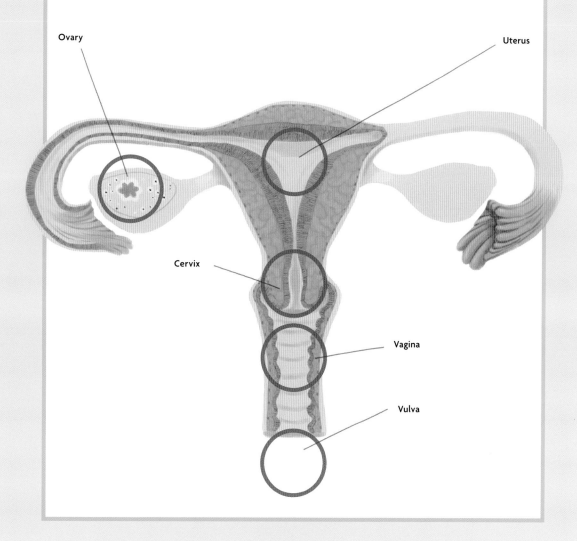

Ovary

Uterus

Cervix

Vagina

Vulva

# Potential gynaecological cancers: what symptoms might warrant a visit to your doctor?

The main symptoms to watch out for are as follows (and just one of these may be a sign of cancer):

- **Abnormal vaginal bleeding** (which is unrelated to your menstrual cycle).
- **Abnormal vaginal discharge** (unlike your usual clear, white odourless secretion).
- **Changes in appetite** – such as feeling full too quickly or loss of appetite – that continue for more than three weeks.
- **Weight loss** that is unexplained by lifestyle changes.
- **Itching, burning, tenderness or sensitivity** in the vulva or vagina.
- **Changes of skin colour** in the vulva.
- **Rashes, lesions, sores or warts** in the vulva.
- **New moles (or changes to existing moles)** in the vulva or vagina.
- **Lumps or bumps** in the vulva or vagina.
- **Pelvic pain** or pressure.
- **Pain and/or bleeding** during or after sexual intercourse.
- **More frequent urgency to urinate** and/or painful urination.
- **Constipation**.
- **Persistent bloating** (for longer than three weeks).
- **Abdominal pain.**
- **Back pain.**

There are some great tools and resources offering gynaecological cancer support online (see Resources from page 241).

## Cervical screening (smear tests)

Millions of women around the world die of cervical cancer each year, so it's really important that you minimize your risk by attending your regular cervical screening appointment. Commonly known as a smear, this test checks for HPV (human papillomavirus) as well as early cervical cell changes and is offered every three years to women aged between 25 and 49, and every five years for those aged between 50 and 65. If you have already had the HPV vaccine (see page 89) you must still attend, as must those who've never had sexual intercourse. This is really important as it is still commonly (and incorrectly) believed that cervical screening is only relevant if you have had sexual contact, and we know that in some cultures pre-marital sex or loss of virginity has a lot of stigma attached to it, which can in turn lead women to avoid having a smear test. If you are a trans or non-binary person with a cervix, and are aged between 25 and 65, you should have a smear test. If you're registered as male with your healthcare provider you may not receive an automatic invite, so check with your surgery that you're listed on their call and recall system.

The smear test takes just a few minutes to perform – either by a nurse or doctor – and patients usually receive their results around two to six weeks later. You may ask for the test to be performed by a clinician of a certain gender (although this isn't always possible) and request a chaperone.

### Preparing for a smear test

It's normal to feel anxious about your cervical screening, especially if it's your first time as the 'fear of the unknown' can be concerning. Please don't let this prevent you from attending this potentially life-saving procedure. Speaking with your nurse or doctor beforehand can be really helpful, since measures can be taken to make smear tests more comfortable. Here are some key points:

- Try to book your smear test at a time when you're not on your period; towards the middle or end of your cycle is ideal.
- Several weeks before your appointment, it's a good idea to start using a topical, water-based vaginal moisturizer to maximize lubrication. You may even want to take some along to the screening.
- Midlife or older women who suffer with vaginal dryness as a result of vaginal atrophy (see page 168), vulvo-vaginal pain or lichen sclerosus (see page 147) may also use topical localized vaginal oestrogen HRT at least one month before their appointment. This medication improves the general health and flexibility of the vaginal walls, which can make the smear test more comfortable. It does not cause or increase the risk of breast cancer, as it gets absorbed directly into the local area as opposed to the bloodstream (it can even be used by women who have, or have had, breast cancer). You can ask your doctor or nurse to prescribe vaginal oestrogen for you in advance.
- You must stop using vaginal oestrogen HRT, oil-based lubricants or spermicides two days before.
- If you have any other physical or psychological concerns – you may have had an episiotomy, for example, or survived FGM or sexual trauma – then please speak to your doctor or nurse beforehand
- Any patients with mobility issues – you may be a wheelchair user, or have severe back pain – may also want to discuss their options in advance.
- If you prefer, you may request a chaperone to accompany you during a smear test; please speak to your surgery beforehand if this is the case.

### What happens at a smear test

As someone who's performed countless smear tests, I can reassure you that it's a safe and simple procedure that should only take a couple of minutes. Here's a run-down of what to expect:

- First of all, you'll be given some privacy and asked to remove your underwear.
- You'll then be asked to lie on a bed with your knees bent, and with your legs open. There may be stirrups into which you can place your heels.
- Once you're comfortable, the nurse or doctor will carefully insert a plastic or metal speculum into your vagina. For ease of passage, they should use a water-based lubricant, which might feel cold at first.
- The speculum is gently inserted sideways, then rotated. Then it is opened up to allow vision and access to the cervix (neck of the uterus). The speculum might make a sound when it is adjusted.
- A long, slender plastic device called a cervix brush, or a swab, is inserted and used to carefully collect the cells on the outer wall of the cervix.
- The brush and speculum are gently removed from the vagina, and you are able to close your legs.
- You'll then be given some privacy to wipe yourself with paper provided, before getting dressed.
- The clinician will place the brush into a sample pot, which will be sent to a laboratory for investigation.

Your comfort should be paramount during a screening – clinicians should do their utmost to make you feel relaxed – but if at any point during your smear test you have any concerns, or do not wish to continue, please make this clear to your healthcare professional. For example, do not be afraid to ask the nurse or doctor, 'Are you using a lubricant on the speculum?' and, if they're not – or don't have any – you have the right to refuse to proceed with the test. You can then ask the surgery to rebook another smear test as soon as possible or to be referred to a specialist clinic (please don't just abandon things, though; you *must* keep that appointment).

Once the test is complete the sample will be sent for testing and you will be told when to expect the results. If no HPV cells are found then no further testing is needed and you should attend your next smear test in three or five years' time. If HPV cells are detected you will either be asked to go for another smear test in a year's time for the doctor to monitor the HPV cells, or you may be referred for a colposcopy, which is a similar process to a smear test and performed in a hospital.

### Preventative care: look after yourself

Cancer is a cruel, indiscriminate disease that can affect people of all ages and backgrounds. It's the cause of one in four deaths in the UK alone, and one in two of us will be affected by it in our lifetimes. In some cases, cancer can be difficult to prevent if you possess an inherited gene. However, in other cases, preventative measures can really help to lessen your chance of getting the disease. I'd be *so* happy if you and your loved ones could consider the following lifestyle changes. They may go a long way towards minimizing your risk, and may help fend off other illnesses, too.

- **Keep your weight down** (preferably BMI below 25).
- **Take regular exercise** (it doesn't have to be strenuous or expensive...120 minutes per week of walking, cycling or yoga is great).
- **Stop smoking** (see page 101).
- **Cut down or cut out alcohol** (women should consume no more than 14 units per week).
- **Minimize stress** (look at ways to reduce anxiety, like listening to music, mindfulness or meditation).

# Having a smear test

The smear test is the routine screening to check the cervix and try to prevent cervical cancer by detecting HPV cells. For the test you will undress from the waist down and the doctor or nurse will insert a speculum (a smooth device) into your vagina. Once in place the speculum is gently widened to allow the doctor or nurse to view the cervix. They then gently wipe a small brush, or swab, over the cervix to collect a sample of cells. Once the sample is collected the speculum will be unwound and removed and you'll be given an opportunity to get dressed in privacy.

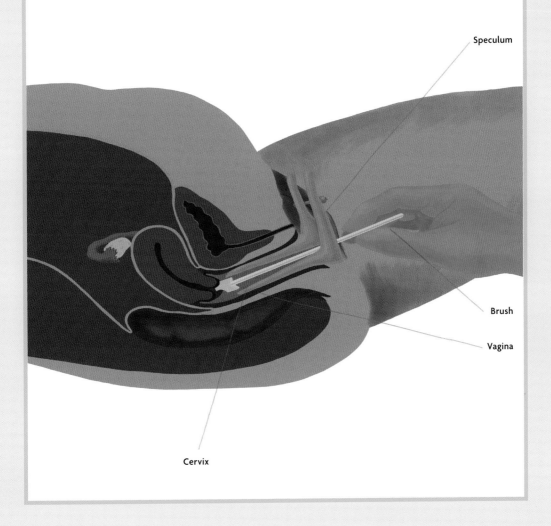

Speculum

Brush

Vagina

Cervix

# Dr Nighat's Takeaways

# 1 Be mindful that things don't always go to plan

If you are planning a pregnancy, give yourself the best chance of conceiving by having unprotected vaginal sex every two to three days.

# 2 If you have had difficulty conceiving for one year...

book a double appointment with your doctor (with your partner if possible) to discuss further investigations.

# 3 Register with the community midwife

As soon as you know you are pregnant, register with the midwife to get your booking appointment. Take folic acid and vitamin D throughout your pregnancy and until you finish breastfeeding.

# 4 Don't miss those screenings

Ensure that you're registered with your healthcare provider for screenings. Make a note of the frequency and call for an appointment if you think you're past due. It's vitally important that you attend, so don't miss out!

# 5 Keep practising self-care!

Examining your own body is crucial in the fight against breast, vulval and vaginal cancer (see pages 16–23 for a full breakdown of self-exmainations). So check your pair, then check down there!

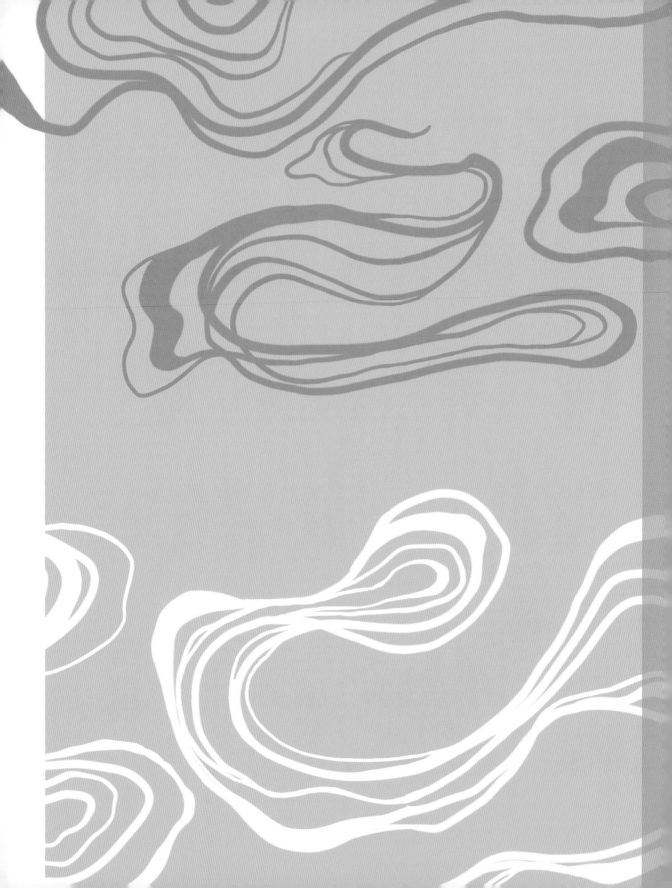

# Your Midlife Years

# Your midlife years: introduction

Midlife — which if the average lifetime is 80 years, has arrived by your forties — should be a time to enjoy and cherish. Maybe your children are no longer getting under your feet, your career is progressing nicely and you have more quality time to spend with loved ones. Perhaps you're feeling full of energy, vigour and optimism, and are ready to embrace the future. If this sounds like you, bravo!

However, for some of us this isn't always the case. As the menopause approaches and our hormone levels naturally plummet, our quality of life can dip. We can begin to suffer problematic symptoms that affect our minds and bodies — from night sweats to vaginal dryness, and from anxiety attacks to memory fog — and, as a result, we're left feeling flat, lost and joyless.

Due to the stigma that surrounds this stage of life — together with an historical lack of knowledge and understanding within healthcare — many individuals opt to suffer in silence rather than seek help. The menopause phase is perceived as something to endure — like menstruation and childbirth — and we should just persevere regardless, perhaps not even realizing that our issues are hormone-related. As a consequence, some women can spend years living with a cocktail of debilitating symptoms, not only receiving limited support or guidance, but also missing out on beneficial treatment.

Luckily, the menopause conversation is starting to change. Awareness of the issue has skyrocketed in the UK over the past few years, largely due to dogged campaigning by healthcare pioneers like Dr Louise Newson, Diane Danzebrink, Kate Muir, Katie Taylor, Nina Kuypers, Dr Annice Mukherjee, Dr Liz O'Riordan, Lavina Mehta, Anita Powell, Meera Bhogal, Dame Lesley Regan, Karen Arthur and Sangeeta Pillai – my heroes! – as well as the sterling efforts of proactive Members of Parliament such as Carolyn Harris, Caroline Nokes and Maria Caulfield. By sharing their midlife stories with such honesty and candour, high-profile TV presenters like Davina McCall, Lorraine Kelly and Louise Minchin have also helped to break the taboo and open the dialogue. Even members of the royal family – the Countess of Wessex being a case in point – are doing their bit to shift attitudes. Menopause is normal and shouldn't be feared!

As a result of this call to arms, an increasing number of women are empowering themselves with menopause-related knowledge, and more healthcare professionals are becoming alive to their needs. I'm so proud to have played my little part in this 'revolution', too – especially within the hard-to-reach ethnic minority community that I hold so dear – and I shall continue to bang my menopause drum on TV and TikTok. Put it this way: I won't be satisfied until everyone in the UK receives the appropriate advice and treatment they need in order to lead the happy and healthy life they deserve.

# The menopause & perimenopause

Everyone who menstruates will experience menopause. In purely medical terms, this is the point in life when you haven't had a period for exactly one year (you're officially deemed post-menopausal the following day). Most women reach this milestone around the age of 52 but, up to a decade prior to that, they're likely to experience what's known as perimenopause.

As women transition through life, their hormones naturally fluctuate. Levels of oestrogen dip significantly as the years pass and the ovaries are gradually depleted of functioning eggs. This perimenopausal phase can trigger numerous changes – there are well over 30 recognized symptoms – which can have a profound effect on a woman's health and wellbeing.

One in four women will sail through the perimenopausal stage without any discernible changes, and will function quite normally on a day-to-day basis. Two in four individuals will experience more significant issues that, to varying degrees, may affect their quality of life, at home, at work and beyond. Sadly, however, one in four women will endure such severe and debilitating symptoms that they'll consider taking their own life: a sobering statistic that never fails to shock me.

Most people start to have perimenopausal symptoms around the age of 40. The National Institute for Health and Care Excellence (NICE) now recommends HRT to reduce hormone-related symptoms such as night sweats and low mood (those aged 40–50 years may need higher doses of oestrogen). HRT will also help to minimize any future risk of osteoporosis and cardiovascular disease, which can be more prevalent among women suffering low oestrogen levels.

As with a woman's menstrual cycle, everyone's menopause is different. There is no one-size-fits-all template. Some women may reach menopause when they're 40, whereas others may do so over a decade later (both are perfectly normal). There's still an awful lot of confusion about the terminology, though; for years, the word 'menopause' has been used as an umbrella term for the whole midlife phase, despite the fact that, from a strictly medical perspective, it only applies to *one day* in a woman's life. The usage of the following definitions is much more accurate:

- **Perimenopause** is when you're still menstruating – even if your periods vary in flow or regularity – and having menopausal symptoms.
- **Menopause** is when you've not had a menstrual period for exactly one year, regardless of any associated menopausal symptoms.
- **Post-menopause** is when you've not had a menstrual period for at least one year and one day, regardless of any associated menopausal symptoms. You will remain post-menopausal for the rest of your life.

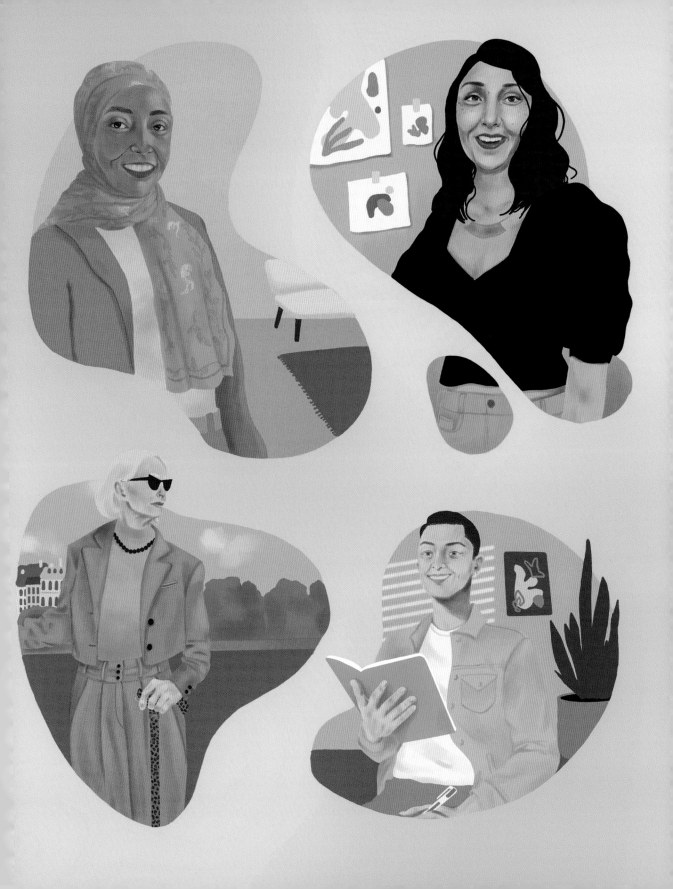

# Early menopause

Early (or premature) menopause (not to be confused with perimenopause) is diagnosed when periods stop before the age of 40. Receiving this diagnosis can be incredibly upsetting and, as fertility is affected, particularly traumatic for those who want to have children.

The causes of reaching the menopause early can be one of the following reasons.

## Premature ovarian insufficiency

Known as POI, this affects one in every 100 women below the age of 40 and occurs when the ovaries stop producing hormones. We're not really sure why POI happens; it may stem from an autoimmune condition, be associated with infections like mumps, malaria and tuberculosis (TB), or there may be a familial link.

Key signs include irregular or missed periods over at least four months, with perimenopausal symptoms (see pages 165–6). A firm diagnosis is usually made after two separate blood tests, performed six weeks apart, show low oestrogen and high follicle stimulating hormone (FSH), but you may also be sent for repeat tests to track your FSH. If you are diagnosed with POI, your doctor will refer you to a gynaecologist for further investigation and treatment. For more information, see Resources from page 241.

## Surgical menopause

Women (or those assigned female at birth) of any age who undergo a total abdominal hysterectomy with removal of the uterus, ovaries, fallopian tubes and cervix, can be plunged into an instant 'surgical' menopause. The removal of the ovaries results in a rapid decline in circulating oestrogen and testosterone, which means the onset of perimenopausal symptoms can be sudden and severe. Prior to surgery, women should be counselled about the risks and benefits of oestrogen-only HRT as it can regulate their symptoms. Younger patients who'd like to have children may also want to discuss the feasibility of harvesting their eggs before surgery, with a view to having children via a surrogate in the future.

Women who only have their uterus removed, and are left with their ovaries intact, are also deemed as being in surgical menopause. However, some of these patients do not realize that they're able to benefit from HRT. Years down the line, they'll come into my surgery suffering with classic perimenopausal symptoms, telling me they thought they didn't need HRT because their ovaries were still working. This can be so frustrating for all concerned.

## Chemical menopause

Chemical menopause is temporary and reversible and can occur when a patient of any age is prescribed a medication called gonadotropin releasing hormone analogues (GnRHa). This drug suppresses ovulation and is used to treat PMDD (see page 64) when less invasive treatments haven't worked. Some cancer treatments, such as certain breast cancer drugs, can also trigger a sudden chemical menopause. If this happens, please initiate a conversation with your doctor or your oncology team about your HRT options.

# Perimenopausal symptoms

Perimenopausal symptoms are such a mixed bag. They can range from the mild to the severe, they can ebb and flow from day to day, and they can affect different individuals in different ways. Some women may experience a handful of symptoms – maybe two handfuls – but others may not notice any changes at all. However, if you recognize any of the tell-tale signs and think you may be perimenopausal, please make an appointment with your doctor. This should ideally be a doctor who specializes in women's health, and/or who has received menopause training; don't be afraid to ask the administration team about this when you ring your surgery.

Perimenopausal symptoms could include any combination of the following:

## Psychological symptoms

- Lack of self esteem
- Lack of self confidence
- Irritability
- Low mood
- Depression
- Lack of libido
- Sleep issues/insomnia
- Forgetfulness/brain fog
- Lack of focus/concentration
- Memory fog/inability to think clearly
- Verbal slips/inarticulacy

## Physical symptoms

- Irregular periods
- Bladder irritation
- Urgent stress incontinence
- Dry skin
- Hair loss
- Digestive problems
- Itchy or watery eyes
- General itchiness (scalp, face, limbs)

- Change in taste
- Change in voice (rasps, wheezes)
- Mouth issues (ulcers, bleeding gums, tooth loss, nerve pain, burning mouth syndrome)
- Tinnitus
- Feeling of skin crawling/electric shocks
- Achy, heavy legs

Keep track of your perimenopausal symptoms so that you feel well-prepared if you need to consult your doctor.

### 'Vasomotor' symptoms

(symptoms relating to blood vessel constriction)

* Palpitations
* Headaches
* Night sweats
* Hot flushes

### Vaginal & vulval symptoms

* Vaginal/vulval dryness (atrophy)
* Vaginal/vulval soreness
* Vaginal prolapse
* Recurrent urinary tract infections (UTIs)
* Difficulty having sex
* Over-lubrication
* Pain when sitting or exercising
* Discomfort during a smear test

You could also refer to the Greene Climacteric Scale (GCS), a measurement tool used by clinicians to assess symptoms with a scoring system. You can find the form online (see Resources from page 241) as it is featured on many menopause-related websites. Take the printout along to your doctor's appointment.

### A note about hypermobility & hypermobility Ehlers-Danlos syndrome in perimenopause

Joint hypermobility is a genetic condition where the joints are more flexible than normal, or the joints move in excess of the normal range of motion. Joints can easily become stiff, and the condition can cause extreme fatigue. Ehlers-Danlos syndrome (EDS) – also known as hypermobility Ehlers-Danlos syndrome (hEDS) – is another genetic condition that, as well as joint-related issues, comprises a collection of symptoms that includes stretchy and/or fragile skin, poor

balance and digestive problems. Many people who suffer with hypermobility and EDS are prone to migraines, but it's not commonly known that all three can be linked to the hormonal fluctuations experienced in perimenopause. If you are diagnosed with these conditions and experiencing perimenopause, the following symptoms can be heightened:

* Brain fog
* Allergies and intolerances
* Joint pain and joint looseness
* Heat intolerance

Fortunately, systemic hormone replacement therapy, or HRT (see page 188), has been shown to improve hypermobility and EDS symptoms – as well as perimenopausal migraine attacks – so, if you are experiencing these symptoms, you may want to discuss this with your doctor.

# 1 in 4 women
## said a lack of support for menopause symptoms in the workplace has made them unhappy in their job

Perimenopause
is a natural
transition that we
should celebrate,
because it means
we made it to our
second spring.

# Vaginal atrophy

Vaginal atrophy, sometimes referred to as vulvo-vaginal atrophy (VVA), is the thinning of the vaginal walls, which can also cause dryness and irritation. It is a common symptom of perimenopuse.

Atrophy literally means 'shrinkage' and occurs when declining oestrogen levels lead to a thinning and loss of elasticity of the vaginal tissue and lining, as well as a reduction of the natural secretions that protect and lubricate the genital area. Low oestrogen levels in the bladder and urethra can also exacerbate recurrent and chronic urinary tract infections (UTIs, see page 72). The bladder is situated extremely close to the vagina and so the condition can affect your bladder, too. These symptoms are particularly worsened for women affected by FGM.

It's thought that around 70 per cent of women (and those assigned female at birth) experience this progressive and chronic condition at some point in their lives. You should definitely not put up with any of these unpleasant symptoms, since effective treatment is readily available.

## Symptoms of vaginal atrophy

- Dry, sore, itchy or inflamed vulva and vagina
- Pain in your bladder and/or urethra
- Recurrent UTIs
- Urgent need to urinate
- Discomfort during urination
- Very painful sexual intercourse
- Discomfort during exercise
- Discomfort and pain when sitting down
- Extreme discomfort during cervical smear test

Symptoms of VVA can range from the mildly irritating to the severely debilitating, and can significantly affect a woman's sexual health and general wellbeing. It is far more common in women over the age of 40 as they approach menopause, but it is also common among women who are breastfeeding. Self examination of the vulva and vagina can really help to pinpoint the issue before you visit your doctor; I've outlined the best way to do this on pages 21–3.

## Diagnosis of vaginal atrophy

Vaginal atrophy is diagnosed by a doctor's examination and discussing your symptoms. Many affected individuals are reluctant to seek help from their doctor, often out of embarrassment or a lack of awareness. Indeed, it's estimated that less than ten per cent of sufferers receive proper care for it, often because they don't realize it's a recognized condition. This is a real shame because, with the right medication, it can be totally manageable.

## Treatment of vaginal atrophy

Targeted treatment for this condition can be genuinely life-changing. People find that vulvo-vaginal itches and inflammation disappear and they go on to have the most pain-free and pleasurable sex ever! Treatments range from non-hormonal to hormonal options and you should discuss with your doctor which are best for you (see page 188).

## Effects of vaginal atrophy

Vaginal atrophy is the thinning and loss of elasticity of tissue in and around the vagina and vulva. It is common in perimenopause as decreasing levels of oestrogen leads to changes to the cells and lining of the vagina. Below the vagina's usual size and thickness is shown on the left and the thinned, less elastic vagina is shown on the right.

**BEFORE**      **AFTER**

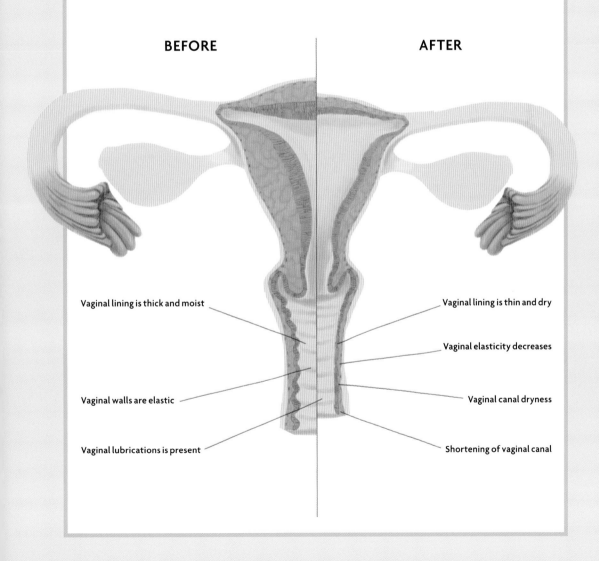

Vaginal lining is thick and moist

Vaginal lining is thin and dry

Vaginal elasticity decreases

Vaginal walls are elastic

Vaginal canal dryness

Vaginal lubrications is present

Shortening of vaginal canal

### Non-hormonal treatments: vaginal moisturizers & lubricants

We regularly moisturize our face, arms and legs to keep the skin plump and supple, so why not give the same TLC to our vulva and vagina, too? Readily available water-based vaginal moisturizers and gels can be used to treat and manage vaginal atrophy, and should be applied to the genital area at least every other day. These can be used during sex, too, as can oil-based vaginal lubricants.

You're never too young or too old to start using vaginal moisturizers. I would advise all women over the age of 30 to get into the habit of regularly moisturizing their vulva and vagina. By doing so they'll be maintaining good health and helping to stave off any future problems. As someone who tries to practise what she preaches, I'm happy to say that I do this at least every other day. Hyalofemme vaginal gel is another option if you prefer a gel formula.

To avoid irritating the vagina or causing infections, I would advise you to ensure your moisturizer or lubricant does not contain glycols, parabens, petroleum, perfume, flavouring, glitter, dyes or tingling ingredients. If you are prone to thrush then also avoid lubricants with glycerins.

### Hormonal treatments: vaginal oestrogen

I am a *huge* fan of vaginal oestrogen – the different types and preparations are listed on page 200–1 – and I could quite literally talk about it all day. It's a simply brilliant treatment for vaginal atrophy and, by restoring urogenital tissues, works to alleviate all those awful symptoms and provide life-long relief. Vaginal oestrogen has no side effects and is completely safe to use, either on its own or in conjunction with other HRT regimes.

Since it contains tiny amounts of hormones (not enough to enter the bloodstream) and just treats the localized vaginal area, vaginal oestrogen does not carry the risks of systemic forms of HRT. It can even be used by patients who currently have breast cancer or who have previously had breast cancer as it does not worsen breast cancer or cause a recurrence. This means that it can be prescribed for women who have (or have had) oestrogen-receptor positive breast cancer. You can also use vaginal oestrogen without progesterone, even if you have a uterus, as the hormone levels are so low.

Some brands of topical vaginal oestrogen act as a lubricant as well as hormonal treatment, therefore they can be used by women whose vulvo-vaginal pain or atrophy may be related to episiotomies, sexual trauma, birth trauma or some cases of female genital mutilation (FGM).

## A note on urinary tract infections caused by vaginal atrophy

Recurrent urinary tract infections (UTIs) are very common during the perimenopause and post-menopause, as they can be exacerbated by declining levels of oestrogen. To tackle these UTIs, women are often prescribed antibiotics by their doctor in the first instance. However, when these infections are frequent, patients can develop a resistance to repeated courses of antibiotics, and this can spiral into life-threatening sepsis. Research has shown that vaginal oestrogen can often be a more effective long-term solution to prevent UTIs from occurring by keeping the vaginal walls plump and lubricated and therefore preventing the irritation that can lead to a UTI.

## External vulval atrophy

Vulval atrophy is the thinning and loss of elasticity of tissue in and around the vulva and usually occurs alongside vaginal atrophy. It is common in perimenopause as decreasing levels of oestrogen leads to changes to the cells and lining of the vulva. Below the vulva's usual size and thickness is shown on the left and the thinned vulva is shown on the right. The thinning and accompanying dryness of vulval atrophy can lead to generalized soreness of the vulva.

**BEFORE**                    **AFTER**

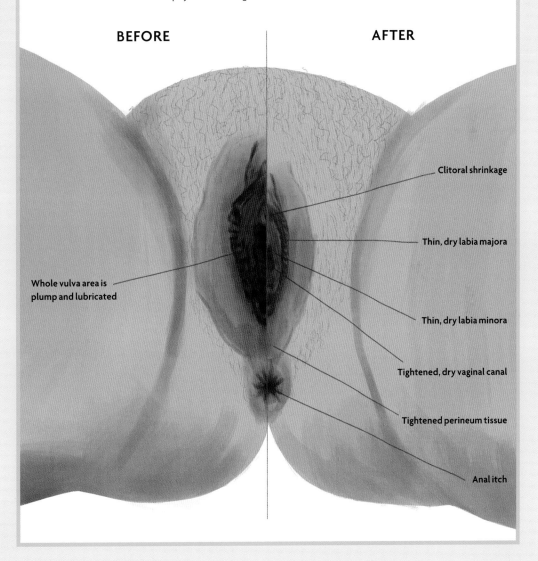

Clitoral shrinkage

Thin, dry labia majora

Whole vulva area is
plump and lubricated

Thin, dry labia minora

Tightened, dry vaginal canal

Tightened perineum tissue

Anal itch

# Urinary incontinence & bladder control

Many women suffer with urinary incontinence and bladder control problems during the menopause phase of life.

Urinary incontinence during menopause is thought to be caused by decreasing levels of oestrogen that may weaken the urethra (the 'tube' that helps keep urine in the bladder until you're ready to pee). The urethra and bladder muscles can also lose some of their strength with the natural ageing process – as is the case with most muscles – and this means you may not be able to hold in as much urine as you get older.

Incontinence can be a very distressing and debilitating condition. It can dominate every thought process, so much so that those affected find themselves planning journeys, work events or day trips based on the location of the nearest toilet. The condition can severely dent a person's confidence and self-esteem, whether it's wearing incontinence pads, worrying about smelling of urine or experiencing leakages during intercourse.

Urinary incontinence impacts one in three women – so if it affects you, you're not alone – and it certainly isn't just an older person's ailment. The condition is not a laughing matter either and, instead of being ridiculed, those impacted should be treated with care and compassion, from doctors recommending tailored treatment to employers offering regular toilet breaks.

### Types of incontinence & their symptoms

- **Urge incontinence** leads to urine leaks when you have a strong urge to wee or when you can't make it to the bathroom in time.
- **Stress incontinence** leads to leaks when you cough, sneeze, laugh or exercise, as these actions increase stress on the bladder and pelvic floor muscles.

### Diagnosis of urinary incontinence

Urinary incontinence is easily diagnosed by keeping track of your symptoms with your doctor.

### Treatment for incontinence

- **Vaginal oestrogen HRT** (see page 190) can improve symptoms of both urge and stress incontinence.
- **Vaginal pessaries** (see page 146) can be prescribed by your doctor to help reduce symptoms of stress incontinence.
- **Medications** can be prescribed to help with incontinence, including solifenacin, tolterodine and mirabegron. These work by relaxing the muscles around the bladder, helping to increase the volume of urine the bladder can hold and control the release of urine.
- **Referral to a urogynaecological specialist** (who can give treatments including Botox™ injections into the bladder) may be possible for some patients, although this is often subject to a postcode lottery.

### Pelvic floor rehabilitation

I recommend that everyone performs 'squeeze and lift' pelvic floor contractions on a daily basis (see page 174) whether or not you suffer with urge or stress incontinence. If you do have symptoms, though, I suggest you gradually try to work towards completing ten long and ten short contractions, three times a day, but if you have no symptoms then once a day is sufficient. Don't over-exert yourself; just take things easy at first, and do what feels comfortable for you. You may also consider reducing your intake of caffeine, alcohol, fizzy drinks and citrus drinks, which are all thought to irritate the bladder.

Ideally, pelvic floor rehabilitation should be done in partnership with a physiotherapist who specializes in that area. You can ask your family doctor for a referral to an NHS physio (who may be based at a local continence clinic) but, again, availability very much depends on your local NHS service provision. Alternatively, you can book yourself in with a private practitioner.

A specialist physiotherapist will tailor a programme of exercises that are right for you, as well as recommending other helpful techniques to help control your bladder leakage. This may include 'the knack' – also known as the counter bracing technique – which is a method of tightly contracting your pelvic floor muscles immediately before a cough, sneeze or laugh.

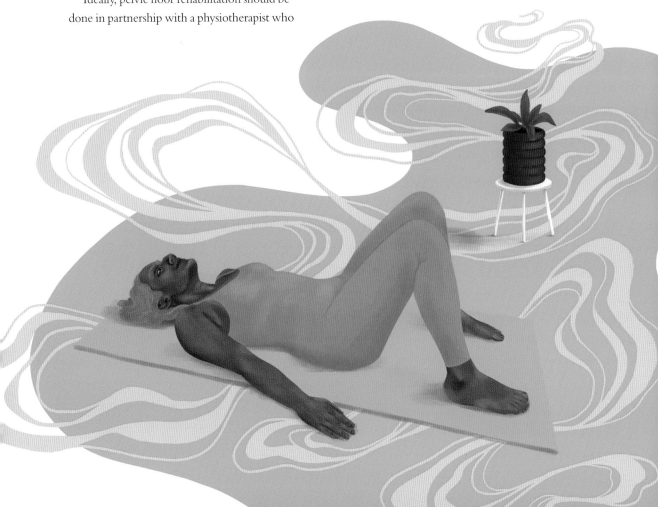

## Pelvic floor exercise

The 'squeeze and lift' pelvic floor contractions shown below will help to tone and strengthen the muscles of your pelvic floor, which in turn can lessen urinary incontinence. Repeat the exercise for ten long contractions (holding each for ten seconds) and ten short contractions (contracting and relaxing in rapid succession), up to three times a day.

**1** Squeeze and lift the muscles at the bottom of your pelvic floor, and at the front and back of your tummy, as if you are trying to hold in urine mid-flow. Hold for ten seconds for long contractions and release immediately for short contractions..

**2** Release the muscles and relax while keeping your posture straight. Repeat these long contractions ten times and then repeat the exercise as ten short contractions.

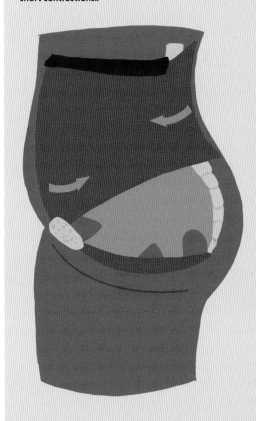

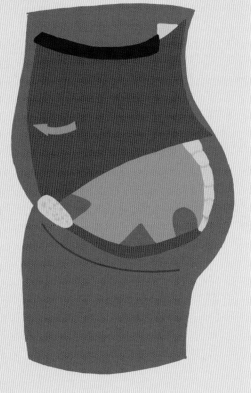

# Perimenopause & contraception: is contraception necessary?

There's a great deal of misunderstanding and misinformation about midlife contraception, so let's first focus on a couple of key facts. Firstly, if you're still having periods – with or without menopausal symptoms – you can still get pregnant. Your eggs can still be fertilized by sperm so you will need to use contraception. Secondly, although some women use the coil as the progesterone element of hormone replacement therapy (see page 202), no other forms of HRT act as a contraceptive! Taking HRT may help to treat your perimenopausal symptoms, but it does not prevent you from becoming pregnant, unless you are using the Mirena™ IUS coil as part of your HRT.

So when can you safely stop using contraception? Here are the guidelines from the NHS:

• **Continue to use contraception for two years** after your last menstrual period if you're under 50 years of age.

• **Continue to use contraception for one year** after your last menstrual period if you're over 50 years of age.

• **Continue to use barrier methods of contraception** (such as condoms) to protect yourself from sexually transmitted diseases, regardless of your age. Contrary to popular belief, STDs can be caught and passed on at any age; according to the charity Age UK, between 2014 and 2018 there was a 23 per cent increase in STD diagnoses among men and women in the 65-plus age bracket.

# Midlife sex issues

There is absolutely no reason why you shouldn't be enjoying a healthy and active sex life well into your middle age (in fact, for the rest of your life). Many patients of mine who are in their forties and fifties will proudly tell me they're having the best sex of their lives, without the inconvenience of monthly periods and the interruptions of young children. Not every woman is so fortunate, however, and many suffer sexual problems that lead them to avoid lovemaking altogether. The hormonal imbalances associated with perimenopause can play a huge part, since they can cause a host of physical and psychological symptoms. If this sounds like you, please don't despair; I'd urge you to talk to your doctor and discuss your options.

## Lack of libido

It can feel awkward and uncomfortable to talk about your sex drive, and most of us won't like to admit that it's in decline. However, low libido is a very common issue among midlife women, and can be treated very successfully. We know that testosterone therapy can work wonders (see page 203) although, at the time of writing, obtaining a prescription can sometimes be tricky as female testosterone is not licensed on the NHS. Testosterone usually prescribed to men can be used 'off licence' in low doses for female HRT use if your NHS doctor has it initiated by a menopause specialist, or feels comfortable prescribing it themselves; the latter usually depends on their local Integrated Care Board (ICB) or Integrated Care System (ICS) marking it as 'green' on their NHS formulary (list of medicines).

There are other non-medical ways to address low libido, too, although they're not necessarily quick fixes. Eating well, minimizing stress and enjoying plenty of exercise can really help things in the bedroom; the latter in particular can boost your levels of serotonin – the so-called 'happy

hormone' – and can make you feel much better about yourself. Patients of mine have often found that, by improving their general wellbeing, their sex life has benefited greatly.

## Sexual dysfunction

A woman's libido can also be affected by any sexual problems her male partner is experiencing. Many men suffer with erectile dysfunction, especially as they approach middle age; this can be linked to underlying issues such as high blood pressure, type 2 diabetes or poor mental health, and often has nothing to do with a lack of intimacy or a lack of sexual chemistry. Nonetheless, erectile dysfunction is still one of those taboo subjects that men and women find really difficult to discuss, even if they've been with their partner for decades. However, as a doctor who's counselled hundreds of couples, I know how common these issues are; statistics show that about 60–70 per cent of couples have sex-related difficulties at some point in their lives. My message to you is, never feel embarrassed to talk to a health professional. Please go and see your doctor – as a couple, ideally – and have that conversation.

## Painful sex

Painful sex can be more prevalent in the menopause phase when women are more likely to suffer with vaginal atrophy. Painful sex is not talked about nearly enough, though – despite being very common – and usually stems from one or more of the following issues:

- Vaginal atrophy or genitourinary syndrome of the menopause (see page 168).
- Vulvodynia (see page 149).
- Endometriosis (see pages 136).
- Birth trauma.
- Female genital mutilation (FGM).
- Vaginismus – this is an autonomic (out of your control) reaction to the fear of vaginal penetration. Whenever penetration is attempted, the vaginal muscles tighten up. You can suffer with occasional vaginismus even if you've had painless vaginal penetrative sex in the past.

*Use lube, lube and **more** lube for each and every vaginal or anal sexual encounter.*

In order to minimize pain and discomfort during sex, I often recommend one of my favourite top tips, namely the double slide method. It takes two to tango in the bedroom, yet so many women – and trans men who still possess a vulva and a vagina – will assume that painful sex is their problem alone. Nothing could be further from the truth...involving your partner is actually part of the solution.

### The double slide method

Before penetration, the woman applies a water-based vaginal moisturizer inside her, which is absorbed into the skin of the vulva and vagina. At the same time, their partner applies an oil-based vaginal lubricant (it has to be vaginal) onto their penis or sex toy.

Find ways of relaxing your body that work for you. Do things at your own pace, communicating what you like to your partner and perhaps showing them yourself. Don't be disheartened if your first attempt at this method doesn't go to plan; try it again on another occasion, but in the meantime keep exploring ways of maintaining intimacy that suit you best as a couple.

The double slide can be really effective due to the fact that oil and water don't mix – they slip and slide – which allows for more comfortable sex. And, since soreness and irritation can be reduced by this method, you're also much less likely to suffer with urinary tract infections (UTIs) which can be very common during perimenopause and post-menopause.

Don't always assume that your anxiety or low mood is symptomatic of depression; it could be the result of a hormonal imbalance.

# Perimenopause & mental health

In midlife, many women notice that perimenopause can have a profound effect on their mental health, mermories and general wellbeing.

Perimenopause can trigger a wide range of psychological symptoms, including the following:

- Memory fog
- Mood swings
- Anxiety attacks
- Lack of motivation
- Loss of confidence
- Paranoid thoughts
- Irritability
- Anger
- Sleep disturbance
- Decreased sexual interest

Some women will also experience suicidal thoughts. Global data suggests that the highest rate of suicide among women is between the ages of 45 and 54, and some studies indicate that this may be related to the biological changes experienced during perimenopause and menopause (see Resources from page 241).

Hormonal fluctuations can wreak havoc with a person's mood, leaving them angry one minute, tearful the next, and confused as to why this is happening. Affected individuals will often say the following when they see me in surgery: 'I can't cope with these meltdowns and mood swings...it's so out of character', 'I feel like I'm losing my mind...I'm so worried I've got dementia', 'I can hardly focus or concentrate on anything...I feel totally lost', 'All the joy has been sucked from my life...I've never felt so depressed'.

This can be a very isolating time, especially if a person believes they're alone in feeling this way. They might also feel an element of shame about their uncharacteristic mood swings and anger, which could deter them from opening up to friends and family. It's very important, therefore, to seek professional help sooner rather than later.

A lack of understanding about perimenopause, however, can lead to misdiagnosis. I've known cases of midlife women being told they're suffering with depression and being prescribed anti-depressants when, in many instances, their emotional and psychological issues are directly related to their changeable hormones, which can be successfully treated and regulated with HRT.

If you experience an acute mental health crisis, and are worried about your immediate safety, call 999 for urgent care.

Other than seeing your doctor, who will be happy to discuss therapies and strategies, there are alternative avenues you can pursue, including:

- **Self-refer to NHS Talking Therapies** (see Resources from page 241)
- **Text 'SHOUT' to 85258** in the UK at time of crisis and a counsellor will text you back.
- **The Samaritans charity** can be contacted by phoning 116123.
- **The Mind charity** can offer support and care for those with mental health issues.

## Neurodiversity during menopause

Neurodiversity refers to a wide spectrum of human behaviour including moods, attention, sociability and learning abilities, and people across the spectrum of neurodiversity should be supported by their healthcare professionals in the best ways for them. All the above behaviours can also, however, be adversely affected by perimenopause, so it can be a particularly disconcerting time for neurodiverse people, and also a time when neurodiverse conditions, that might have been missed in earlier life, may be diagonosed.

Autism, attention deficit hyperactivity disorder (ADHD), Tourette syndrome and dyslexia are common neurological conditions and people with autism and ADHD in particular can notice a significant impact on their mental wellbeing during perimenopause.

### Autism spectrum disorder

Throughout a person's lifetime autism spectrum disorder (ASD) can affect communication, behaviour, social skills, attentiveness and learning. There is currently very little research into the effects of perimenopause on individuals with ASD, but on the few studies that we do have, the common denominator indicated a significant increase during perimenopause in autism-related symptoms, such as socializing, communicating and sensory sensitivity.

Data also shows that women are generally better at 'masking' their symptoms and finding coping strategies to deal with ASD and so women have historically been underdiagnosed in comparison to men. This has had a knock-on effect in the lack of studies around the effects of ASD during perimenopause.

### Attention deficit hyperactivity disorder

Commonly known as ADHD, this is a common condition diagnosed in both children and adults, that manifests in hyperactivity, difficulties paying attention and impulsive behaviour.

The reduced oestrogen levels associated with perimenopause also reduce levels of dopamine, a chemical that aids executive functioning. This means that women with ADHD can find their symptoms worsened by the hormonal changes of perimenopause, in addition to the common mental health implications of perimenopause.

One survey, by *ADDitude* magazine, found that more than half of the women surveyed said 'ADHD had the greatest impact on their lives' during the perimenopausal years from their forties to their fifties with brain fog and memory issues having the most impact. In addition, many women also report ADHD symptoms for the first time during perimenopause. If you are diagnosed with ADHD, discuss your HRT options with your doctor, as oestrogen replacement could have a significant impact on your wellbeing.

# Lifestyle changes to help relieve perimenopausal symptoms

In midlife, many women make lifestyle changes to control their perimenopausal symptoms but these will have a huge beneficial effect on their overall wellbeing, too.

## Sleep

Cognitive behavioural therapy (CBT) can help with sleep issues by encouraging positive thoughts and better habits (see pages 186–7) but there are other practical things you can also do to aid a restful night:

- **Avoid eating meals late at night**, and steer clear of alcohol and caffeine.
- **Take a bath** before you go to bed.
- **Keep your bedroom cool**, dark and ventilated.
- **Place a towel beneath you** to absorb perspiration and protect your sheets.
- **Use a special cooling pad pillow** (there are plenty on the market), which can ease night sweats.
- **Wear loose cotton nightwear** that can easily be removed in bed.
- **Reduce distractions before bedtime**; maybe read a book or listen to calming music rather than watch TV or scroll social media.
- **Use a sleep app** to help you dose off (see Resources from page 241).

## Diet

Maintaining a varied and nutritious diet can make a significant difference to your general health and wellbeing, and this is particularly important as you approach the menopause. Many individuals in this phase of life find themselves gaining weight – especially around their abdomen – which is often the result of the following factors:

- Fluctuating hormone levels can affect the way your body stores fat, leading to fewer calories being burned, and more fat building up.
- A decrease in muscle mass means your body may crave more calories, and you may end up eating more food than you actually require.
- You may be less inclined to take regular exercise because of perimenopausal symptoms such as insomnia, fatigue, hot flushes and joint pain.

Weight gain in the midlife years can often increase your risk of certain illnesses – such as type 2 diabetes and cancer – so it's vital that you watch what you eat and drink. I'm no fan of restricted, prescriptive diets – I much prefer sensible, achievable and balanced healthy eating plans – and my key advice to patients is as follows:

## Eat lots of fruit & vegetables

Fruit and veg should form a core part of your daily diet. My esteemed colleague Dr Mary Claire Haver, a US-based obstetrics and gynaecology physician who specializes in women's nutrition, recommends eating a 'rainbow' of brightly coloured fruit and veg. So that means plenty of orange satsumas, red grapes, green peppers and purple sprouting broccoli!

### Up your intake of fibre & protein

Make sure your daily food quota includes lots of high-fibre, starchy carbohydrates (such as brown rice, wholegrain pasta and baked potatoes) as well as a variety of protein-rich foods such as oily fish, lean meat, eggs, nuts, seeds and legumes (beans and pulses).

### Cut down on highly processed food & junk food

Try to reduce your intake of processed foods, takeaways and ready meals. They may contain high levels of salt and saturated fat, and can lack essential nutrients. Some cured meats may also contain a preservative called sodium nitrate that has been linked to cancer and heart disease.

### Eat sugary foods only in moderation

I'm not averse to grabbing a slice of cake or a bar of chocolate when I'm feeling tired or stressed. However, while I don't deny myself the occasional treat, I try not to make it a daily habit. Foodstuffs with added sugar such as sweets, cakes, biscuits and fizzy drinks – as well as those with hidden sugars, like pasta sauces and flavoured yogurts – should be consumed in moderation.

### Reduce portion sizes

Your stomach is much smaller than you think – it's actually about the same size as your clenched fist (go on, try it!) – so try reducing your portion size accordingly. To prevent overeating, learn to recognize the feeling of your stomach being full, and remind yourself that you don't have to clear the entire plate.

### Maintain good gut health

It's so important to keep your gut healthy. Not only does it detoxify and eliminate what we consume, it also controls our mind and body. It's responsible for managing neurotransmitters such as serotonin (the 'happy hormone'), dopamine, cortisol and melatonin, all of which affect our mood and sleep. The gut also plays an integral part in the menopause phase. We know that oestrogen, together with other hormones and toxins, gets excreted into the gut before being eventually eliminated from the body via faeces. Constipation is common in the perimenopause and post-menopause, however, and if the gut microbes become imbalanced it can lead to oestrogen absorbance dominance. This can heighten menopausal symptoms, hence why you need to look after your gut by sticking to a healthy and nutritious diet.

### Consider food supplements & vitamins

In order to maintain healthy joints, skin and hair during menopause – and to look after your

**81.9%**
of postmenopausal women have low levels of magnesium

immune system – I generally recommend the following dietary supplements to my patients:

- Vitamins $B_6$, $B_7$ (biotin) and $B_{12}$
- Vitamin D
- Magnesium
- Collagen
- Zinc
- Calcium
- Omega 3 oil
- Evening primrose oil
- Soya isoflavones

Some of the above can be found in multivitamin tablets (which I recommend you take on a daily basis in any case), but others may need to be purchased separately.

### Eat phytoestrogens

There is also some evidence to suggest that foods high in phytoestrogens – including olive oil, soya beans, tofu, miso, liquorice root tea, beans, pulses, oats, nuts and seeds – can relieve symptoms of hot flushes and can improve bone health.

### Cut down on alcohol

Not only does alcohol contain 'empty' calories, it can also worsen common perimenopausal symptoms like hot flushes, night sweats and low mood. Excessive consumption also increases your risk of cancer and heart disease, among other illnesses. If you can't eliminate it altogether, stick to the NHS recommended limit of 14 units of alcohol per week.

> Healthy eating habits, drinking plenty of water, getting regular exercise and good-quality sleep can make such a difference to perimenopausal symptoms. Give yourself time for some self-care!

### Drink plenty of water

I can't stress how important water is. Not only does it quench your thirst, it also helps to regulate your body temperature, lubricate your joints, ease your digestion, improve concentration and stave off infections. Staying well hydrated also aids a good night's sleep. The NHS Eatwell guide suggests we drink six to eight glasses of fluid per day; some of this quota can include decaffeinated tea, low-fat milk and sugar-free drinks.

## A note on making changes to your diet

Anyone with special dietary requirements (such as those with coeliac disease or type 1 or type 2 diabetes) should always talk things through with their doctor before changing their eating regime.

## Exercise

Keeping yourself fit is essential as you transition towards menopause, and is crucial for your long-term health. Regular physical activity at this stage in life helps to:

- Build muscle.
- Strengthen bones.
- Control stress and anxiety levels.
- Boost mood and mindset.
- Lower blood pressure.
- Increase metabolism.
- Maintain a healthy weight.
- Promote social interaction.

I recommend a minimum of 25 minutes of exercise, five days a week. Ideally, this should comprise a combination of resistance training – with free weights or fixed weights – and weight-bearing and cardiovascular, workouts such as running, walking, swimming or dancing. This regime can also be complemented with regular stretching, strengthening and breathing exercises, such as those practised in yoga or pilates. Now I know it can feel difficult to fit exercise into a busy life, but remember that every little helps. I like to pepper my day with exercise 'snacks', and have listed a few ideas on the right to get you started.

Osteoporosis is an incredibly debilitating condition, and can severely affect your quality of life. I know patients in their sixties and seventies suffering with poor bone strength who struggle to walk short distances, who are unable to carry their grandchildren, and who can't even lift themselves up off the toilet. So that's why it's massively important to consider your long-term health and put measures into place before it's too late. You will also find some exercise-related resources in the Resources section from page 241.

### EXERCISE 'SNACKS'

- Get off the bus or train a couple of stops early and finish your journey with a brisk walk.
- Jump off the sofa and try doing a few squats while you're watching TV.
- Exercise your pelvic floor muscles with a quick 'squeeze and lift' movement whenever you stop at traffic lights.
- Clench and release your buttock muscles while you wait in line for your morning coffee.
- Try a few push-ups off the kitchen counter while you're waiting for the kettle to boil.
- Use time that you're catching up with friends and family on the phone as an excuse to get out walking, or ask a colleague to switch a regular meeting into a 'walk and talk' session instead.

## Histamine intolerance

Histamine is a compound that is released by cells all over our body and works on our nerves to produce itching. Histamine intolerance happens when our immune system mistakenly believes that a harmless substance is actually harmful to the body.

Histamine intolerance is an issue that's only recently entered the menopause arena, and it's really piqued my interest. So what is it, exactly? Well, oestrogen is an immune modulator – a substance that helps support the immune system to fight disease and infection – and, if it goes into decline, your immune system thinks it's under attack and over-produces histamine.

### Symptoms of histamine intolerance

- Bloating
- Headaches
- Nausea
- Rashes and itchiness

Histamine intolerance means your system is unable to sufficiently break down the excessive histamine. Added to this, it is believed (but under-researched) that levels of the digestive enzyme diamine oxidase (DAO) are reduced during perimenopause, which further exacerbates histamine intolerance so that some women suddenly find themselves unable to tolerate certain foods. The worst culprits are foods that contain high levels of 'biogenic amines' (amino acids that are released when fermentation takes place) such as processed meat, canned fish, fermented vegetables, mature cheese and red wine.

Conversely (and confusingly) some women who are given oestrogen HRT also experience a surge in histamine levels – sparking similar reactions to those detailed opposite – which, again, we think occurs as the body tries to defend itself.

### Diagnosis of histamine intolerance

Histamine intolerance is not a well-known condition and currently diagnosis is simply through the discussion of symptoms with your doctor. However, midlife women – as well as their doctors – will often mistake symptoms of histamine intolerance for an allergic reaction, pure and simple, when in fact the underlying trigger is more likely to be hormonal. You can measure DAO activity in the blood serum histamine level, but this is not currently available on the NHS.

### Treatment of histamine intolerance

People who've just started HRT can be justifiably alarmed to experience these symptoms – some even consider stopping their treatment – but I would urge you to hang fire and talk to your doctor as there are a number of treatment options:

- **Reduction of histamine-rich foods in your diet**, which would take 14 days to deduce a difference. (I am not endorsing an elimination diet here, but be mindful of what foods cause a reaction for you.)
- **Low-dose antihistamines** such as cetirizine or loratadine – commonly used as hay fever remedies – can be taken to counteract symptoms (I often recommend a three-month course of 10 milligrams per night), after consultation with a medical professional.
- **The anti-nausea drug stemetil** can also be beneficial after consultation with a medical professional.
- **Changing your dose of systemic HRT** (or moving to topical vaginal HRT only), but think carefully about the wider benefits that you may risk losing, too.

# Complementary & alternative therapies

The perimenopause is a perfectly normal transition in life, when your periods stop and your oestrogen and progesterone levels are declining. Many women take an holistic approach to their health during this phase, using alternative therapies on a stand-alone basis or to complement more conventional treatments. They might also reassess their lifestyle, perhaps cutting down on alcohol, taking more exercise and trying to reduce their stress at work.

As an NHS doctor, I have no qualms chatting about alternative remedies in my clinic – I use a few of them myself – but I'm also mindful that there can be a lack of evidence-based research surrounding them. While I'm happy to help navigate patients around the various options – and signpost them to relevant resources – it's ultimately up to them to find out what suits them best, from mindfulness and meditation to reiki and reflexology (see Resources from page 241).

Being an NHS doctor, I can't endorse complementary therapies to my patients. However, I'm happy enough to be told anecdotally that something is easing their menopause symptoms. The following therapies are most often cited in my surgery.

## Acupuncture

Acupuncture – the ancient Chinese practice of inserting thin needles into the body – is reported to lower hot flushes and night sweats. See Resources from page 241 to help you find an accredited therapist.

## Herbal treatments

Herbal therapy has grown in popularity over the years, and I've known many women who swear by Korean ginseng, red clover, black cohosh or St John's wort to manage their perimenopausal symptoms. However, it's very important that these therapies are taken with care, as they can interfere with other medicines. Women on tamoxifen (a post breast cancer hormone-suppressing treatment) should avoid St John's wort, for example, and, in some cases, black cohosh has been known to cause liver toxicity. To ensure that you're taking a regulated product, check for the Herbal Register Stamp before you purchase. See Resources from page 241 to help you find an accredited practitioner.

## Cognitive behavioural therapy

Cognitive behavioural therapy (CBT), according to the NHS, is 'a talking therapy that can help you manage your problems by changing the way you think and behave'. Indeed, the National Institute for Health and Care Excellence (NICE) now recommends it as a therapeutic option to alleviate feelings of stress, anxiety and low mood that can be experienced during perimenopause,

menopause and post-menopause. Some patients greatly benefit from it – either via self-help, or by working with a qualified specialist – but others find it pretty fruitless and ineffective; it can be a tricky concept to grasp, and needs a lot of practice and application. Like many elements of menopause treatment, there's no one template that suits everybody; it really is a case of 'each to their own'.

Cognitive and behavioural strategies such as breathing exercises and managing your thought processes are known to help with hot flushes. This common menopausal symptom can be quite embarrassing and uncomfortable for those who experience it, especially when it happens in public. Paced, controlled breathing, in which you relax your body and breathe from your stomach, can be really beneficial, as can learning how to manage your feelings when that tell-tale flush engulfs you.

CBT can also help with sleep issues. Many perimenopausal women suffer with insomnia – often worsened by night sweats – yet this can often be controlled by changing your bedtime behaviour and restructuring your thought patterns. This might involve deploying some relaxation techniques, or removing certain sleep distractions (including putting that pesky mobile phone in a drawer!).

CBT is widely available on the NHS everywhere, especially in light of the pandemic, as part of the government's Every Mind Matters initiative. Alternatively, you can try CBT on a self-help basis, without being referred by your doctor (see Resources from page 241).

If you are on HRT, you should always tell your doctor if you're taking complementary medicines.

## Acceptance & commitment therapy

An increasing number of my patients with menopausal symptoms, particularly hot flushes, are practising acceptance and commitment therapy (ACT), although it's not yet available on the NHS. At its core, ACT is a mindfulness-based therapy that encourages you to accept your situation as it is, rather than fighting against it, which may sometimes mean learning to take the rough with the smooth. An ACT therapist will also help you to commit to tackling issues head on, rather than avoiding them, and will also teach you to manage your negative thoughts.

# Hormone replacement therapy

There are myriad ways to tackle perimenopause and menopause and minimize symptoms, and as a healthcare professional it's my job to look at each person, assess their situation and connect the dots. A patient can have hormonal treatments and/or non-hormonal treatments – all have pros and cons, and risks and benefits – and during the first consultation, we will work closely together to ascertain how best to manage symptoms. Going down the non-hormonal route is often my first starting point, which generally involves embracing an holistic approach to diet, exercise and lifestyle (see pages 181–4). That being said, many of my patients have already tried those lifestyle changes before they come to see me.

For those individuals whose symptoms are not improved by this non-hormonal course of action, and whose quality of life is still suffering as a result, hormone replacement therapy (HRT) can be a fantastically beneficial treatment. HRT doesn't suit everyone – and I never pressure a patient to take it – but as a doctor who's successfully issued it to hundreds of patients, I can bear witness to its transformative effects.

## How HRT works

HRT is simply a supplementation of the hormones that are lacking in a woman's body as she transitions towards the menopause. It consists of two hormones that I've mentioned often in this book – oestrogen and progesterone – and, in some cases, can incorporate a third hormone, testosterone. Women (and those assigned female at birth) who have a uterus will ordinarily use a combination of oestrogen *and* progesterone – this is to prevent the thickening of the endometrial lining of the uterus, which can be caused by oestrogen-only treatment. But those who've had a hysterectomy will usually take oestrogen by itself.

Hormone replacement therapy is designed to relieve a whole host of troublesome perimenopausal symptoms including palpitations, insomnia and depression (see pages 165–6 for the full list). Studies suggest it may have long-term benefits, too, including a reduced risk of osteoporosis, dementia, type 2 diabetes, depression and cardiovascular disease.

HRT is available on prescription in a variety of preparations and combinations and, depending on the woman's individual needs, some types can be adjusted and fine-tuned on a day-to-day basis. This is ideal for women who have cyclical symptoms which vary in intensity. HRT is also available as 'systemic HRT' – tablets, patches or gels that treat symptoms throughout the body; or 'topical HRT' – creams, gels and pessaries that only treat symptoms in the genitals.

By seeking help and guidance from your doctor – and by allowing yourself time and patience to discover your best 'fit' – you can benefit from a bespoke HRT regime to control your hormones and ease your symptoms. What's not to love?

### Using HRT

HRT is usually offered to three groups of patients:

* **Those showing classic perimenopausal symptoms** who wish to relieve the symptoms.
* **Those who experience premature ovarian insufficiency** (POI), surgical menopause or chemical menopause (see page 164).
* **Those with perimenopausal symptoms** who want to protect themselves against osteoporosis and other conditions such as heart disease and vascular dementia.

I choose not to apply an upper or lower age limit when I prescribe HRT, simply because the needs of my patients are paramount. They may be 43, or 53, or 63, but if they're sitting in my surgery, struggling with a litany of tell-tale symptoms, I'll gladly discuss the pros and cons of HRT.

Unlike other medications, HRT is not given as a course of treatment and, if it aids a woman's health and wellbeing, there's no reason why it can't be taken indefinitely (essentially for the rest of a woman's life). HRT does not delay menopause – that's a question I'm often asked – but simply controls symptoms while they are present.

Minor side effects are common in the first few weeks of HRT treatment – such as nausea, leg cramps and breast tenderness – so I often advise my patients to persevere during these early stages. Once everything has settled down, any side effects can be minimized by adjusting HRT types and doses.

In my experience, women wait until their symptoms get really bad, about four years, before going on systemic HRT. It doesn't have to be this way! Don't wait until your symptoms get severe before plucking up the courage to talk about HRT with your doctor.

**Over $1/3$ of women who visited their doctor with perimenopausal symptoms were offered antidepressants**

## HRT treatment formats

There are a few different ways to take HRT:

- **Oral tablets and capsules** are usually taken daily so they are easy to remember. Oestrogen tablets are associated with a slightly higher risk of clots than patches or gels, because they are processed by the liver. They can also lower libido and may not be suitable if you are obese or have certain health conditions. They can be less reliable in terms of absorption if you have an upset stomach.

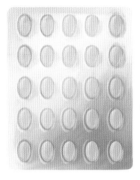

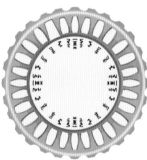

- **Skin patches** are stuck onto the skin and changed once or twice a week. These give a constant dose so can be good if you suffer from migraines. You can also use multiple patches if you need a higher dose. The adhesive used can leave a sticky residue, but that can be easily removed with baby oil.

- **Skin gels and sprays** are usually rubbed over your arms or legs. They make it easy to control the dose so your doctor can tailor a very specific dose according to your requirements or advise you to use them in conjunction with a patch. They can ease PMS symptoms if you still have periods, and the dose can be increased for the days before your period if necessary.

- **Implants** are inserted by a healthcare practitioner and can be useful for women who do not absorb oestrogen well. However, they can lead to fluctuating hormone levels and doses are less flexible than in other formats.

- **Vaginal pessaries and creams** are only used topically. Creams are applied around the vulva, vagina, bladder, urethra and perineum, for symptoms associated with the lowering of oestrogen levels in the body, while pessaries are inserted into the vagina.

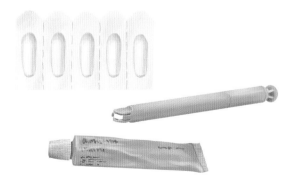

## HRT treatment types

The best HRT treatment for you depends on your personal circumstances. In general, they can be classified as one of the following:

- **Combined HRT** contains both oestrogen (which relieves menopausal symptoms) and progesterone (which reduces the risk of oestrogen causing abnormal changes to the lining of the womb). If you still have periods (whether monthly or irregularly), you would usually take the oestrogen element continually and the progesterone element for two weeks in every four. If you are post-menopausal, you would take the treatment continually.

- **Oestrogen-only HRT** is suitable if you have had a hysterectomy. People who have had a hysterectomy do not usually need to include progesterone in their HRT as there is no risk of their oestrogen treatment causing abnormal changes to the lining of the uterus (since it has been removed). However, if you've had a hysterectomy as a result of severe endometriosis, then your doctor might want to include a progesterone supplementation in case there are any endometrial cells left in the pelvis. Similarly, if a hysterectomy didn't include removal of the cervix, then in some cases women might also need progesterone as part of their HRT to prevent any remaining endometrial cells from thickening abnormally. Oestrogen-only HRT can also be taken by those who have not had a hysterectomy if taken alongside a progesterone-only HRT. This can work well for women who find they have unwanted side effects from certain oestrogens or progesterones.

- **Topical vaginal oestrogen** suitable for women who suffer the effects of vaginal atrophy (see page 168). As it is topical, it does not carry the associated risks of other forms of HRT and is therefore suitable for women who have, or have had, oestrogen-receptor positive breast cancer. Topical vaginal oestrogen does not relieve systemic menopausal symptoms.

## Body identical HRT

Due to medical and scientific advances, there's a growing list of HRT preparations. The latest, newer-generation treatments are particularly brilliant; they're known as body identical, which means they mimic the chemical shape and structure of our own natural hormones. They are plant-based, and I find myself recommending them, rather than the older-generation, synthetic types of HRT, more frequently. The transdermal body-identical oestrogens – gels, sprays and patches – are perceived as particularly safe options since they're absorbed through the skin rather than being processed by the liver. Body-identical progesterones are also derived from plant-based ingredients, and studies have shown they have fewer risks and side effects than their synthetic counterparts (see page 209). Weighing things up with a medical practitioner will help you decide if the body-identical route is best for you.

### Beware compound bio-identical hormones

You may come across references to 'compound bio-identical' hormones, but they should *not* be confused with 'body-identical' hormones. These are in fact unregulated medicines, often marketed as 'natural', that are prescribed privately by specialist clinicians. Neither NICE nor the British Menopause Society (BMS) believe these 'bio-identical' products have enough robust data to demonstrate their safety and efficacy (please check out the BMS website if you'd like to read more).

## Cyclical combined HRT

✓ Suitable for women with a uterus, who have perimenopausal symptoms
   and still bleed
✓ In a typical cycle, combined oestrogen and progestogen tablets are taken for two
   weeks in every four and oestrogen-only tablets are taken for two weeks in four

| PRODUCT NAME | OESTROGEN TYPE + PROGESTOGEN TYPE | SYNTHETIC (S) OR BODY-IDENTICAL (B)? | DELIVERY | NOTES |
|---|---|---|---|---|
| Elleste Duet | estradiol + norethisterone acetate | S | oral tablets | • Taken daily so easy to remember<br>• Slight increase in risk of clots<br>• Less reliable absorption than transdermal forms<br>• May not be suitable if you are obese or have type 2 diabetes<br>• First line oral treatment option for most healthcare practitioners |
| Femoston | estradiol hemihydrate + dydrogesterone | S | oral tablets | • Taken daily so easy to remember<br>• Slight increase in risk of clots<br>• Less reliable absorption than transdermal forms<br>• May not be suitable if you are obese or have type 2 diabetes<br>• Offered as an alternative if the norethisterone progestogen in Elleste Duet causes side effects, such as erratic bleeding patterns, acne or dizziness |
| Prempak C | conjugated oestrogens + norgestrel | S | oral tablets | • Taken daily so easy to remember<br>• Slight increase in risk of clots<br>• Less reliable absorption than transdermal forms<br>• May not be suitable if you are obese or have type 2 diabetes<br>• Made from mare's urine, which can deter patients |

| | | | | |
|---|---|---|---|---|
| **Evorel Sequi** | estradiol hemihydrate + norethisterone acetate | B | transdermal patches | • Adheres to the thigh or buttock and can be worn in the bath, shower or while swimming<br>• Offers a constant dose of oestrogen<br>• First line transdermal option for most healthcare practitioners |
| **FemSeven Sequi** | estradiol + levonorgestrel | B | transdermal patches | • Adheres to the thigh or buttock and can be worn in the bath, shower or while swimming<br>• Offers a constant dose of oestrogen<br>• Can be used as an alternative if patients have skin allergies, poor absorption or poor adhesion with other patches |
| **Personalized bespoke option** | oestrogen of choice + progesterone of choice (most commonly Utrogestan capsules taken cyclically or the Mirena™ IUS coil) | depends on formats chosen | depends on formats chosen | • Can be used if you experience side effects (such as bleeding problems) from the progesterone types used in other combined treatments |

* Always consult your own doctor before starting any new treatment.

## Continuous combined HRT

✓ Suitable for women with a uterus, who have not had a period
for more than 12 months

✓ The combined oestrogen and progestogen tablets are taken continually

| PRODUCT NAME | OESTROGEN TYPE + PROGESTOGEN TYPE | SYNTHETIC (S) OR BODY-IDENTICAL (B)? | DELIVERY | NOTES |
|---|---|---|---|---|
| Kliovance | estradiol + norethisterone acetate | S | oral tablets | ◆ Taken daily so easy to remember<br>◆ Slight increase in risk of clots<br>◆ Less reliable absorption than transdermal forms<br>◆ May not be suitable if you are obese or have type 2 diabetes<br>◆ First line oral treatment option for continuous HRT |
| Femoston Conti | estradiol hemihydrate + dydrogesterone | S | oral tablets | ◆ Taken daily so easy to remember<br>◆ Slight increase in risk of clots<br>◆ Less reliable absorption than transdermal forms<br>◆ May not be suitable if you are obese or have type 2 diabetes<br>◆ An alternative if there are side effects (bloating or tender breast tissue) with other progestogens |
| Premique low dose | conjugated estrogens + medroxyprogesterone acetate | S | oral tablets | ◆ Taken daily so easy to remember<br>◆ Slight increase in risk of clots<br>◆ Less reliable absorption than transdermal forms<br>◆ May not be suitable if you are obese or have type 2 diabetes<br>◆ Usually offered if you have reacted well to cyclical equine oestrogen previously<br>◆ Made from mare's urine, which can deter patients |

| | | | | |
|---|---|---|---|---|
| **Indivina** | estradiol + medroxyprogesterone | S | oral tablets | • Taken daily so easy to remember<br>• Slight increase in risk of clots<br>• Less reliable absorption than transdermal forms<br>• May not be suitable if you are obese or have type 2 diabetes<br>• Offered if you have had bleeding on other forms of continuous combined HRT and uterine pathology has been ruled out (including polyps, fibroids, thickening of endometrial lining) |
| **Angeliq** | estradiol + drospirenone | S | oral tablets | • Taken daily so easy to remember<br>• Slight increase in risk of clots<br>• Less reliable absorption than transdermal forms<br>• May not be suitable if you are obese or have type 2 diabetes<br>• Can be used as an alternative if there are side effects with other progestogen types (such as bloating, acne or tender breast tissue) |
| **Tibolone** | tibolone (a synthetic molecule with oestrogen, progestogen and androgenic properties) | S | oral tablets | • Taken daily so easy to remember<br>• Slight increase in risk of clots<br>• Less reliable absorption than transdermal forms<br>• May not be suitable if you are obese or have type 2 diabetes<br>• The androgenic properties been found to improve low libido in some studies<br>• Can also be considered post hysterectomy and/or bilateral salpingo oophorectomy (BSO) |

continues overleaf

| | | | | |
|---|---|---|---|---|
| Bijuve | estradiol hemihydrate + progesterone | S + B | oral capsules | • Taken daily so easy to remember<br>• Less reliable absorption than transdermal forms<br>• Unlike other oral tablets, this is more suitable for women who have clot and migraine history because it contains body-identical micronized progesterone<br>• The risk of breast cancer is lower in younger women compared with oral synthetic continuous combined HRT |
| Evorel Conti | estradiol hemihydrate + norethisterone acetate | B + S | transdermal patches | • Adheres to the thigh or buttock and can be worn in the bath, shower or while swimming<br>• Offers a constant dose of oestrogen<br>• First line treatment for transdermal continual HRT<br>• Patches applied twice a week |
| FemSeven Conti | estradiol hemihydrate + levonorgetrel | B + S | transdermal patches | • Adheres to the thigh or buttock and can be worn in the bath, shower or while swimming<br>• Offers a constant dose of oestrogen<br>• Can be used as an alternative if patients have skin allergies, poor absorption or poor adhesion with other patches |
| Personalized bespoke option | Oestrogen of choice + progesterone of choice (most commonly Utrogestan capsules taken continually or the Mirena™ IUS coil) | depends on formats chosen | | • Can be used if you experience side effects (such as bleeding problems) from the progesterone types used in other combined treatments |

* Always consult your own doctor before starting any new treatment.

In my clinical experience, there is NO individual who cannot have treatment in some form to help relieve menopausal symptoms, even those who have (or have had) cancer.

## Oestrogen-only HRT

✓ Suitable for women who've had a hysterectomy (so have no uterus)

✓ Suitable for women who still have a uterus but want to take progestogens separately

| PRODUCT NAME | OESTROGEN TYPE | SYNTHETIC (S) OR BODY-IDENTICAL (B)? | DELIVERY | NOTES |
|---|---|---|---|---|
| Elleste Solo | estradiol | S | oral tablets | • Taken daily so easy to remember<br>• Slight increase in risk of clots<br>• Can lower libido<br>• Less reliable absorption than transdermal forms<br>• May not be suitable if you are obese or have type 2 diabetes |
| Premarin | conjugated estrogens | S | oral tablets | • Taken daily so easy to remember<br>• Slight increase in risk of clots<br>• Can lower libido<br>• Less reliable absorption than transdermal forms<br>• May not be suitable if you are obese or have type 2 diabetes<br>• Made from mare's urine, which can deter patients |
| Evorel | estradiol | B | transdermal patches | • Adheres to the thigh or buttock and can be worn in the bath, shower and while swimming<br>• Offers a constant dose of oestrogen |
| Elleste Solo Mix | estradiol hemihydrate | B | transdermal patches | • Adheres to the thigh or buttock and can be worn in the bath, shower and while swimming<br>• Offers a constant dose of oestrogen<br>• Can be used as an alternative if other patches cause skin allergies, or have poor absorption/ adhesion |

| | | | | |
|---|---|---|---|---|
| **Estradot** | estradiol hemihydrate | B | transdermal patches | • Adheres to the thigh or buttock and can be worn in the bath, shower and while swimming<br>• Offers a constant dose of oestrogen<br>• Available in smaller-sized patches with a higher concentration of active ingredients, so more suitable for higher doses and petite women |
| **Sandrena** | estradiol hemihydrate | B | transdermal gel (sachet) | • Very easy to use<br>• Simple to regulate dosage if symptoms are cyclical<br>• Can be used as an alternative if patches cause skin allergies<br>• Individual sachets are less environmentally friendly than other options |
| **Oestrogel** | estradiol hemihydrate | B | transdermal gel (bottle) | • Very easy-to-use and a highly popular option with patients<br>• The 100ml bottle can be taken in hand luggage<br>• Simple to regulate dosage if symptoms are cyclical<br>• Can be used as an alternative if patches cause skin allergies<br>• Plastic bottle can be recycled<br>• Can be subject to shortages |
| **Lenzetto** | estradiol hemihydrate | B | transdermal spray | • A very light, easily absorbed preparation that is sprayed onto skin<br>• Simple to regulate dosage if symptoms are cyclical<br>• Can be used as an alternative if patches cause skin allergies<br>• Currently more expensive in comparison to other formulas so some doctors may be reluctant to prescribe |

* Always consult your own doctor before starting any new treatment.

# Topical vaginal oestrogen

✓ Suitable for women with symptoms relating to genito-urinary syndrome of the menopause, which includes dryness, burning, itching, painful sex and recurrent UTIs

✓ Vaginal oestrogen does not ease other perimenopause/menopause-related systemic symptoms

| PRODUCT NAME | OESTROGEN TYPE | DELIVERY | NOTES |
|---|---|---|---|
| Vagifem | estradiol | vaginal pessary | ◆ Self-administered in a single-use applicator<br>◆ A number of treatments are usually required<br>◆ Use one pessary every night for 2 weeks and then reduce to 2–5 times a week, settling on the frequency that relieves your symptoms<br>◆ Safe for women with breast cancer on Tamoxifen |
| Vagirux | estradiol | vaginal pessary | ◆ Self-administered with a reusable applicator<br>◆ A number of treatments are usually required<br>◆ Use one pessary every night for 2 weeks and then reduce to 2–5 times, settling on the frequency that relieves your symptoms<br>◆ Safe for women with breast cancer on Tamoxifen<br>◆ Suitable for women with a past history of breast cancer, who are not currently on AI or Tamoxifen, if Estring is not tolerated |
| Imvaggis | estriol | vaginal pessary | ◆ Very low dose format<br>◆ Highly lubricated and easy to insert<br>◆ Self-administered with a reusable applicator<br>◆ A number of treatments are usually required<br>◆ Use one pessary every night for 2 weeks and then reduce to twice a week, although guidelines allow up to 5 times a week at your doctor's discretion. |
| Gina | estradiol | vaginal pessary | ◆ Available over the counter in the UK, for women over the age of 50 who have not had a period for at least one year and who have vaginal menopausal symptoms<br>◆ Self-administered with a reusable applicator<br>◆ A number of treatments are usually required<br>◆ Use one pessary every night for 2 weeks and then reduce to 2–5 times, settling on the frequency that relieves your symptoms |

* Always consult your own doctor before starting any new treatment.

| Gynest/ Estriol/0.01% | estriol | vaginal cream | <ul><li>Self-administered with a reusable applicator</li><li>Some find a cream more comfortable to insert than a pessary</li><li>A number of treatments are usually required</li><li>Use one dose every night for 2 weeks and then reduce to twice a week, although guidelines allow up to 5 times a week at your doctor's discretion.</li></ul> |
|---|---|---|---|
| Ovestin | estriol | vaginal cream | <ul><li>Self-administered with a finger or a reusable applicator</li><li>Can be applied externally to just the vulva as well as internally into the vagina</li><li>A number of treatments are usually required</li><li>Use one dose every night for 2 weeks and then reduce to twice a week, although guidelines allow up to 5 times a week at your doctor's discretion.</li></ul> |
| Generic creams | estradiol | vaginal cream | <ul><li>A number of generic creams are available on prescription</li><li>Self-administered with a finger or an applicator</li><li>These can be oily so are not condom-friendly and can be messy</li><li>They can contain peanut oil unsuitable for those with an allergy</li><li>The length of time that effects last varies according to the brand</li></ul> |
| Estring | estradiol | vaginal ring | <ul><li>This flexible ring is inserted in a similar manner to a tampon</li><li>Can be fitted yourself or by your doctor</li><li>Effects last for 3 months per insertion, so it is useful and effective for women who can't manage daily use themselves</li><li>You can leave it in to have sex or it can be removed if needed</li><li>Good alternative if you find yourself using Vagifem or Vagirux at the maximum established dose of five times a week</li><li>Safe for use by women who have had, or currently have, breast cancer on Aromatase Inhibitors (AI, such as Anastrozole or Exemestane), because it provides a constant slow release of topical oestrogen, rather than loading 2 or 3 times weekly</li><li>First line for women with a past history of breast cancer, who are not currently on AI or Tamoxifen</li></ul> |
| Blissel | estriol | vaginal gel | <ul><li>Self-administered with a reusable applicator</li><li>Highly hydrating and non-greasy</li><li>A number of treatments are usually required</li><li>Use one dose every night for 2–3 weeks and then reduce to twice a week, although guidelines allow up to 5 times a week at your doctor's discretion.</li><li>Slightly more expensive than other products so doctors may be reluctant to prescribe</li></ul> |
| Intrarosa DHEA/ Parastone DHEA | DHEA (an androgen that converts into an estrogen when in the body) | topical pessary | <ul><li>Self-administered with a reusable applicator</li><li>Inserted into the vagina once daily at bedtime</li><li>Highly hydrating and non-greasy</li><li>A number of treatments are usually required</li><li>Safe to use for patients who have had, or currently have, breast cancer and are on aromatase inhibitors (such as Anastrozole or Exemestane)</li></ul> |

## Progestogens & progesterones

✓ Suitable for women with a uterus who do not want to take a combined HRT treatment

✓ Progesterone on its own does not relieve perimenopausal/menopausal symptoms but is used in combination with an oestrogen-only treatment to reduce the risks of oestrogen-only treatment

| PRODUCT NAME | PROGESTERONE/ PROGESTOGEN TYPE | SYNTHETIC (S) OR BODY-IDENTICAL (B)? | DELIVERY | NOTES |
|---|---|---|---|---|
| Utrogestan | progesterone | B | oral capsules | • Cyclical regime for women who are menstruating: 200mg at bedtime for 2 weeks out of 4<br>• Continuous combined regime for women whose periods have stopped for a year: 100mg at bedtime, daily<br>• The oral capsules can also be taken vaginally (at half the oral dose, at the discretion of your menopause specialist) to avoid side effects, such as bloating, acne, dizziness, low mood or other progesterone intolerance symptoms |
| Provera | medroxyprogesterone acetate | S | oral tablets | • Cyclical regime for women who are menstruating: 10mg at bedtime for 2 weeks out of 4<br>• Continuous combined regime for women whose periods have stopped for a year: 2.5–5mg at bedtime, daily |
| Intrauterine system (Mirena™ IUS coil) | levonorgestrel | S | coil inserted into uterus by clinician | • Also acts as a contraceptive<br>• Can stop heavy periods<br>• Insertion can be painful and initially cause erratic bleeding<br>• Each coil lasts for 5 years for HRT use, after which it can be renewed |
| Cyclogest/ Lutigest | progesterone | B | vaginal pessary | • Commonly used as part of fertility treatments<br>• If they are experiencing progesterone intolerance, some women prefer to use these (off licence at the discretion of your menopause specialist) |

\* Always consult your own doctor before starting any new treatment.

## A note about stopping sequential/ cyclical HRT regimes

Some patients ask me when they should stop taking progesterone cyclically, and transfer over to a continuous regime. If you're on a combined sequential/cyclical regime that contains oestrogen and the progesterone-only mini-pill, your fertility is suppressed, so you won't have periods and therefore won't be able to gauge when you're medically menopausal. So, if you're under the age of 45 your doctor will need to stop your HRT regime for four weeks before giving you two blood tests, six weeks apart, to check your levels of oestrogen and follicle stimulating hormone (FSH) in order to establish whether you're menopausal and need to change your regime. But if you're above the age of 45, your doctor won't deem it necessary to perform a blood test and will just switch you over to continuous HRT.

If you're on a combined sequential/cyclical regime that consists of an oestrogen-only product taken alongside progesterone, your fertility is not suppressed, so you will still be menstruating. However, once your periods reach a natural cessation – and you don't experience a bleed for 12 months – you'll be deemed menopausal and will be switched over to continuous HRT.

## A note about the progesterone coil & progesterone-only pill

If you have a progesterone coil or are taking the progesterone-only pill and are not having periods, and are wondering 'Am I in the menopause?', you can seek help from your doctor. If you're over the age of 45, you'll probably not need a blood test; your doctor will diagnose you by your symptoms alone. Women under the age of 45 can be given

'off licence' refers to using medication in a way that's not typically recommended by the manufacturer. It does not make the suggested usage clinically unsafe as is commonly practiced under the guidance of doctors and other medical professionals.

the FSH test, and your doctor may also check for issues such as anaemia and thyroid function, liver and kidney function.

## Testosterone

There's been a lot of debate around testosterone. Contrary to popular belief, testosterone is not just a male preserve; women actually need it, too. It contributes to libido, orgasm and sexual arousal, and plays a vital role in maintaining urogenital health, muscle and bone strength, skin collagen levels and cognitive function. It's a hormone that has many roles to play and, whenever we talk about HRT treatment for menopausal symptoms, it should definitely form part of that conversation.

If your doctor is treating you for low sexual desire with testosterone therapy, it is important that urogenital tissues are adequately treated with vaginal oestrogen (see page 170) to avoid painful or uncomfortable sex.

Testosterone can be taken alongside an oestrogen and progesterone HRT regime, and is usually a gel-based treatment that is easily rubbed onto the skin. However, this hormone should only be prescribed by a doctor like myself who is specially trained in testosterone therapy for low sexual desire, once a bio-psychosocial approach has excluded relationship issues, stress, and anti-depressant medications such as SSRIs or SNRIs (see page 213).

As I write, there is no uniformed way of prescribing testosterone in the UK. Other countries, including Australia, willingly prescribe this hormone to women, so why can't we? The Aussies have even produced a female-specific preparation (Androgel/Androfeme, see page 205) so I can only assume that they attach more value to a woman's sex life than the Brits!

While it's possible for a patient to receive testosterone treatment, getting a prescription isn't always straightforward. More often than not, the patient's symptoms alone will tell the story and will allow the clinician to make a sensible diagnosis, but when they request testosterone, they will have to undergo a blood test to measure their base levels of androgens – a group of sex hormones – and to check that there aren't any other underlying and treatable reasons for any deficit.

Testosterone isn't an instant fix – it can take a few months for a person to notice any clinical difference – but, when it does kick in, the effects can be remarkable. Patients of mine have reported a massive increase in their sex drive and their general wellbeing, which is a pretty wonderful outcome for all concerned!

As of October 2022, the British Menopause Guidelines state that for all testosterone products, your total testosterone level should be checked before treatment begins. After six weeks of use, an additional test is required to assess effectiveness. Once on an established dose, monitoring continues every 6–12 months to ensure that the levels remain within the female physiological range.

However, if a patient hasn't noticed any difference after six months, the British Menopause Society (BMS) guidelines suggest that the testosterone treatment should be stopped, and other management avenues should be explored.

## Testosterone treatments

✓  Suitable for women with low libido

✓  Can also contribute to good urogenital health, and help muscle and bone strength and cognitive function

| PRODUCT NAME | DELIVERY | NOTES |
| --- | --- | --- |
| Androfeme | transdermal cream | • The only testosterone cream that is currently licenced for use in women in the UK<br>• Can take several months to work<br>• Frequency of use is at the discretion of your menopause specialist<br>• Synthesized from soya so not suitable if you have an allergy |
| Androgel | transdermal gel | • The only testosterone gel that is currently licenced for use in women in the UK<br>• Can take several months to work<br>• Frequency of use is at the discretion of your menopause specialist<br>• Synthesized from soya so not suitable if you have an allergy |
| Testogel | transdermal gel | • Licenced for use in men; can be used off licence to provide female physiological testosterone replacement<br>• Available in sachets<br>• Can take several months to work<br>• Frequency of use is at the discretion of your menopause specialist |
| Testim | transdermal gel | • Licenced for use in men; can be used off licence to provide female physiological testosterone replacement<br>• Available in a canister<br>• Can take several months to work<br>• Frequency of use is at the discretion of your menopause specialist |
| Tostran | transdermal gel | • Licenced for use in men; can be used off licence to provide female physiological testosterone replacement<br>• Available in a canister<br>• Can take several months to work<br>• Frequency of use is at the discretion of your menopause specialist |

* Always consult your own doctor before starting any new treatment.

# The risks of hormone replacement therapy

There are potential risks for some women taking HRT, as there are with most medical treatments, so it's important to arm yourself with the facts before embarking on treatment. However, I believe that all women can find something suitable for their level of risk and current situation to help their symptoms.

Not every woman is a candidate for HRT when the risks can potentially outweigh the benefits, and as doctors we look at individual symptoms as best we can. If you're considering HRT, you need to discuss your own particular circumstances with your doctor so request a double appointment if you can. Your age, lifestyle, medical history and personal preference will be taken into account.

For the majority of women who are prescribed HRT, I believe the pros considerably outweigh the cons. I, like many of my colleagues, believe that the newer, body-identical HRT products not only effectively manage the symptoms of perimenopause, but can also lessen the risk of conditions such as osteoporosis, vascular dementia and heart disease. Preventative care is the core principle of the NHS, when all is said and done, and I think HRT perfectly fits that purpose. Indeed, since 2019, the guidance from the National Institute for Health and Care Excellence (NICE) is clear that HRT should be recommended as a first-line therapy to perimenopausal women to help symptom control and to aid future health.

There are some risks with HRT and, if you want to find out what's best for you, you need to discuss the pros and cons with your doctor face-to-face and, if possible, arm yourself with evidence-based research (see Resources from page 241).

All I would say, though, is that I've known some individuals who are eligible for HRT but, being fearful of the risks, decide against using it and continue to suffer horrendous perimenopausal symptoms. So my message is: please don't deny yourself HRT without thoroughly exploring the upsides and downsides.

*As regards HRT, always ask yourself, 'Do the benefits outweigh the risks?'*

**IMPORTANT!
We need to stop
scaring women
about oestrogen,
and instead
empower them
with evidence-
based information.**

# Understanding the risks of breast cancer

**Women's Health Concern**

A confidential independent service for women and their partners

A comparison of lifestyle risk factors versus hormone replacement therapy treatment.

**Difference in breast cancer incidence per 1,000 women aged 50–59.**
Approximate number of women developing breast cancer over the next five years.

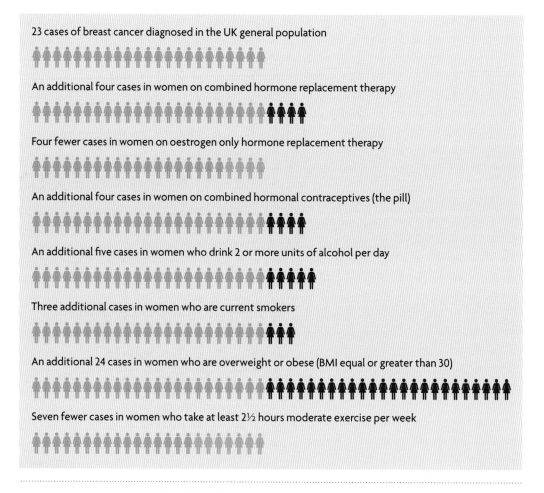

23 cases of breast cancer diagnosed in the UK general population

An additional four cases in women on combined hormone replacement therapy

Four fewer cases in women on oestrogen only hormone replacement therapy

An additional four cases in women on combined hormonal contraceptives (the pill)

An additional five cases in women who drink 2 or more units of alcohol per day

Three additional cases in women who are current smokers

An additional 24 cases in women who are overweight or obese (BMI equal or greater than 30)

Seven fewer cases in women who take at least 2½ hours moderate exercise per week

**Women's Health Concern**

**Women's Health Concern is the patient arm of the BMS.**
We provide an independent service to advise, reassure and educate women of all ages about their health, wellbeing and lifestyle concerns.

Go to **www.womens-health-concern.org**

**BMS**
British Menopause Society

Q2P2223

## Breast cancer & HRT

Breast cancer (see pages 222–4) is a life-changing disease that affects millions of women across the globe. Although it is commonly linked to old age those in younger age groups, or those assigned female at birth with breast tissue, can also contract it. In the UK, one in seven women will develop the disease at some point in their life.

In the past, some clinical studies have linked breast cancer with HRT. The infamous Women's Health Institute study in the early 2000s, for example, which received huge coverage in the media, claimed that synthetic, systemic oestrogen – now regarded as one of the 'older' types of HRT – significantly increased the risk of breast cancer and heart disease. This turned out to be a misleading assertion, closer inspection of the study data showed this heightened risk wasn't solely related to oestrogen. There was a slight increase in women developing breast cancer if they used combined synthetic oestrogen *and* synthetic

> Self examination of the breasts and breast tissue (at all ages), is the best way to pick up early breast changes.

progesterone HRT, but this amounted to just one in every 1,000 women per year.

However, more recent studies – including a paper entitled 'Menopausal hormone therapy formulation and breast cancer risk', published in June 2022 by the American College of Obstetricians and Gynaecologists – have made it clear that breast cancer risks are comparatively lower among individuals using the new-generation, body-identical versions of HRT. Opposite is a graphic that I find hugely helpful, courtesy of the BMS, showing the breast cancer risks of HRT versus other factors.

The key facts are as follows:

- Women below the age of 50 using HRT comprising transdermal, body-identical oestrogen and micronized progesterone have a lower relative risk of breast cancer, in comparison with the older version of HRT.
- Women below the age of 50 who've had a hysterectomy (and therefore use transdermal, body-identical oestrogen on its own) do not have an increased risk of breast cancer.
- Women over the age of 50 who choose to take HRT for menopausal symptoms will have a slightly higher risk of breast cancer than those who do not take HRT, but remember: the older you are, the higher your risk is anyway.
- There is no increased risk of breast cancer among women who take vaginal oestrogen to relieve menopausal symptoms (even if they have, or have had, breast cancer).
- Thanks to improved breast screening, far fewer women in the UK are dying from breast cancer nowadays. Screening mammograms – together with the urgent cancer referral system – are helping with early detection and better prognosis.

But fears about oestrogen still linger, despite growing evidence that suggests it does not cause breast cancer alone. As clinicians, we *have* to emphasize to our patients that this is the case, and we need to explain that the wider picture is far more multi-layered. Family health history, biological female status, advancing age and possession of breast tissue will naturally increase the risk of developing breast cancer, as might lifestyle choices relating to diet, exercise, smoking and alcohol. Indeed, according to Cancer Research UK, having a BMI above 30 increases your chances of breast cancer by 50 per cent in women over the age of 50. Drinking two or more glasses of wine per night (or exceeding the recommended amount of 14 units of alcohol per week) proves to be riskier than taking the newer, body-identical types of HRT.

That said, by suggesting that breast cancer can often be related to lifestyle, age or genetics, I do not wish to alienate, aggravate or in any way 'blame' sufferers and survivors. I sometimes receive kickback online from individuals who feel my observations are unfair, especially if their own health and wellbeing regime has been exemplary, but – along with many other menopause specialists – I just believe that, in general, the benefits of HRT outweigh any potential risks.

I also appreciate that some individuals feel discriminated against because they're unable to take HRT due to a cancer diagnosis, or because of other illnesses or conditions. I am very conscious of this and, whether it's in my surgery or on social media, I'm happy to recommend alternative medical treatments (see page 213) and complementary and alternative therapies (see pages 186–7) that may benefit those patients.

## Blood clots & HRT

Studies show that transdermal oestrogen, unlike synthetic oral oestrogen, does not increase the risk of blood clots, known medically as venous thromboembolism (VTE). Also, compared with synthetic progesterones, micronized progesterone shows a reduced risk of clots when used in combination with oestrogen. This means that patients who have migraines, who are overweight, who have a family history of clots (or have had a clot in the past that has been treated) can be considered for body-identical HRT, subject to the risks and benefits being weighed up for each individual patient.

Like all sex hormones, oestrogen is derived from cholesterol, so patients who already have high cholesterol levels or who have underlying heart disease need to be careful when taking oral HRT containing estradiol (a type of oestrogen). We have a background risk of having clots due to estradiol in our bodies. Hence the increased risk of clots with the combined oral contraceptive pill as that also contains estradiol. However, taking transdermal oestrogen as a patch, gel or spray – when it's absorbed through the skin – does not increase your background risk of clots.

## Heart disease, strokes & HRT

Transdermal, body-identical oestrogen, as opposed to oral synthetic oestrogen, does not increase cardiovascular risk. Micronized progesterones and dydrogesterone (which are both body-identical) also have a neutral effect on your cholesterol levels, your glucose metabolism and your blood vessel tone. This means, therefore, that your risk of strokes and heart disease is lower when taking body-identical HRT, compared with the synthetic versions.

It is important to note that if you have breast cancer or have had breast cancer, you can still have topical vaginal oestrogen HRT for vaginal dryness or genitourinary syndrome of menopause.

### Endometrial cancer & HRT

The risk of endometrial cancer is greatly reduced in women who have a uterus when oestrogen is given in combination with progesterone. The progesterone can be supplied via oral capsules, a patch or a coil. If a woman has a uterus, and is using micronized progesterone administered vaginally (albeit off licence), it may actually improve endometrial protection. This is because it works at the uterus level and bypasses liver metabolism, therefore protecting against endometrial cancer when using oestrogen.

And, while we're on the subject of uteruses, a quick note about HRT and endometriosis: hormone replacement therapy can be taken by women with a history of endometriosis (this includes testosterone). However, individuals who've had a hysterectomy should be advised that oestrogen treatment can potentially reactivate some of their endometriosis symptoms. To combat this, they may be offered a little bit of progesterone or continuous HRT to help manage their symptoms. So, if you're an endometriosis sufferer who no longer has a uterus, please don't be deterred from taking HRT if you are experiencing menopausal symptoms; instead, chat through your options with your doctor.

### Ovarian cancer & HRT

There is no increased risk of ovarian cancer in women with a uterus who take combined, systemic oestrogen and progesterone. Studies show that taking oestrogen on its own very slightly increases the risk of ovarian cancer, so oestrogen-only therapy is only given to women who've had a hysterectomy or have no uterus. If a woman has had her uterus removed but still has ovaries, she will also be given oestrogen-only therapy because a progesterone element to prevent thickening of the uterus is not needed. In this instance therefore, the small increased risk of ovarian cancer will remain.

### Weight gain & HRT

There is a common misconception that HRT can cause weight gain but there is no data to show this to be the case. In fact, studies show that HRT helps you to manage a healthy weight because of improved energy levels and better sleep, which provides added motivation to exercise and follow a healthier diet.

# HRT supply & shortages

The upsurge in demand for HRT is a beautiful thing, in my opinion – it signifies that more and more women are taking control of their own hormones – but in recent years it's led to serious shortages and supply issues, particularly with the newer body-identical products. This causes a great deal of worry and stress for all involved – thousands of women are reliant on oestrogen – it also prompts clinicians like myself to question whether the problem would be allowed to escalate if there was a country-wide shortage of insulin for those with type 1 diabetes or Viagra™. To me, it is yet another example of a patriarchal healthcare system effectively devaluing women's healthcare needs.

I've read a few articles effectively blaming the media for HRT supply issues, and maligning doctors for over-prescribing it. This is a ridiculous standpoint. We should be celebrating the fact that legions of women are benefiting from HRT, not bemoaning it. You'll certainly never catch me apologising for signing off a stack of prescriptions for oestrogen and progesterone, that's for sure. Empowering a woman to make the right choices for her long-term health and wellbeing will always be my priority.

If you're faced with shortages and need to substitute your regular HRT, it's really important that you discuss this with your doctor. Absorption can vary between preparations, and there may be an element of trial and error before you find the level that works. This table provides a guide for oestrogen products, which most commonly see shortages, but the British Menopause Society (BMS) also advises on equivalent doses for progesterone, see the Resources section from page 241.

| Body identical HRT: equivalent doses of oestrogen products | | | | |
|---|---|---|---|---|
| Patch | Half a 25 microgram patch | 25 micrograms | 50 micrograms | 75–100 micrograms |
| Gel – pump | Half a pump | 1 pump | 2 pumps | 3–4 pumps |
| Gel – sachet | Half a 0.5 milligram sachet | 0.5 milligram sachet | 1 milligram | 1–2 milligrams |
| Spray | N/A | 1–2 sprays* | 2–3 sprays* | over 3 sprays* |

* These are approximate doses. Absorption of the spray can be very variable, with many individuals finding they need to use large quantities for symptomatic benefit. Always consult your own doctor before starting any new treatment.

# Other prescribed treatments for menopausal symptoms

Not all perimenopausal and post-menopausal people will pursue the HRT route. For some this is out of their control since they may suffer with medical conditions that prevent them from taking it. For others this is out of choice as they may simply want to try different options. The good news is that there are plenty of alternative treatments to consider, many of which are non-hormonal and can be prescribed by your doctor. I'm always happy to discuss all the whys and wherefores with my patients, and I'm sure your own doctor will be, too.

## Gabapentin

This anticonvulsant medicine can help to combat hot flushes and night sweats. Its mechanism for alleviating these specific conditions is unknown, but we think it works on the hypothalamus, the section of the brain that regulates temperature. It does have side effects, though – especially if it's taken in higher doses – which include drowsiness, dizziness, weight gain and a dry mouth. It's a controlled drug that needs to be prescribed by your doctor, but please note that it may not be suitable for those who have stage three or four kidney disease, chronic obstructive pulmonary disease (COPD) or have an allergic reaction to gabapentin.

## Pregabalin

This anticonvulsant and anti-anxiety medication can be prescribed, in low doses, to help with hot flushes. Side effects can include sleepiness, dizziness, headaches and blurred vision, and it's not recommended for patients who suffer with suicidal thoughts, COPD, chronic kidney disease or an existing addiction to pregabalin.

## Clonidine

This non-hormonal drug is often used to treat high blood pressure (some brands are used for attention deficit hyperactivity disorder/ADHD) and is also licensed to help prevent hot flushes. Studies have shown that it is effective in this respect, but that it doesn't help with any other menopausal symptoms. One of its side effects is drowsiness, so it may well aid sleep and prevent insomnia. As it's an anti-hypertensive drug, I would not usually prescribe this to someone with low blood pressure.

## Anti-depressants

Anti-depressant medications, such as selective serotonin reuptake inhibitors (SSRI) or serotonin-noradrenaline reuptake inhibitors (SNRI) are available on prescription and can really help with perimenopausal symptoms, primarily hot flushes. Side effects can include nausea, drowsiness, dizziness, headaches, blurred vision and low sex drive; doctors may not recommend SSRIs or SNRIs to anyone who has previously suffered side effects from them, or who is addicted to anti-depressants.

# Menopause happens to women of all creeds, cultures and ethnicities!

# Menopause in Black, Asian & ethnic minority communities

Menopause remains a taboo subject within ethnic minority communities which, by nature, tend to be very reserved and inhibited. I know from experience that many women in South Asian communities abide by a cultural attitude known as *purdah* – keeping things 'under the veil', in other words – which hinders discussion about gynaecological issues such as menstruation and menopause. These perfectly natural processes are deemed as dirty and unseemly – or are sometimes even sexualized – which leads to many women glossing over symptoms and suffering in silence, just to spare their blushes.

In addition, some of my patients regard the menopause as a Western phenomenon that only affects Caucasian women, and will often dismiss any tell-tale physical symptoms they experience themselves such as headaches, joint pain and vaginal atrophy. They may also gloss over emotional and psychological issues such as anxiety, paranoia, low mood or low self-esteem for fear of being seen as *pagal*, or mad. Others who are able to withstand sweltering temperatures in Delhi or Dubai will often play down vasomotor symptoms (related to blood vessel constriction) such as hot flushes or night sweats when they are back home in the UK, telling themselves they are mild in comparison and don't merit a doctor's appointment.

This whole mindset is really concerning because it means that women aren't benefiting from effective, life-changing treatment. When you hide things 'under the veil' you miss out on preventative healthcare, you're unable to benefit from treatment and, as a consequence, you can't pass on your knowledge and experience to others. People from South Asian, Middle Eastern and Black communities are particularly prone to type 2 diabetes, heart disease and osteoporosis as midlife approaches, and starting them on HRT before the age of 60 may actually reduce the risk of these complications, as well as improving their perimenopausal symptoms.

On average **women of colour experience perimenopause earlier** than their white counterparts and experience perimenopausal symptoms for longer

This situation can be exacerbated by the systematic discrimination that still exists within the healthcare sector, including a worrying lack of research relating to menopause and women of colour. However, while there's much work to do on these fronts, things are gradually improving. More Black and South Asian women than ever before are proudly telling me that they're receiving treatment for their menopausal symptoms, which makes my heart sing!

## Menopause & Ramadan

Contrary to popular belief, Muslim women *can* continue to take all forms of HRT while fasting during the holy month of Ramadan. I've worked with the Royal College of Obstetricians and Gynaecologists, Muslim Women UK, and Imam Allama Arif Hussain Saydee MBE to produce guidelines for those who fast, but if you are concerned, you may also want to discuss things with your scholar.

The following types of HRT are not classed as having any nutritional qualities, so are perfectly permissible to use during Ramadan:

- **Transdermal oestrogen patches, gels and sprays** can be taken during Ramadan. The fact they're adhered or applied to your thigh or upper arm means that the hormones are absorbed through the skin, and head straight into your muscle and fat cells. You are not therefore breaking your fast. However, if you're using a gel or spray that needs to be applied manually on a daily basis, you may prefer to do this at the time of *sehri/suhoor* (before sunrise, so before you start fasting) or *iftar/iftari* (after sunset, when you break your fast).

- **Progesterone capsules** can be taken at *iftar*, once you've broken your fast. They should only be taken at night-time in any case, and they have the added benefit of helping you sleep.

- **A Mirena™ IUS coil** is inserted into the uterus so is not classed as nutritional, and does not break your fast.

- **Vaginal oestrogen** helps with genitourinary syndrome of the menopause (GSM), which can include conditions such as vaginal dryness and painful sex. Because it is applied topically – directly onto the affected area – it can be used during Ramadan and does not affect your fasting. Again, you may prefer to apply the cream or insert pessaries after *iftar*, following your evening prayers.

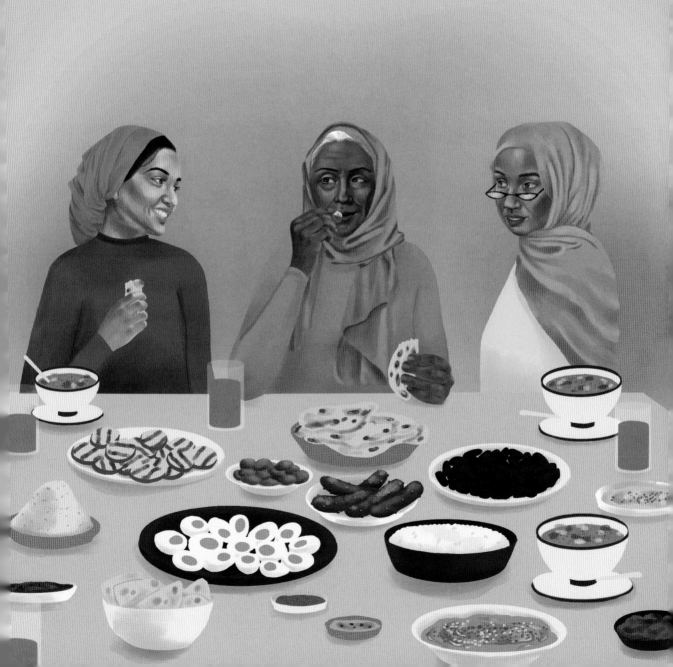

# Approaching your doctor about menopause

Women are far less likely to seek help with perimenopausal symptoms compared with other more obvious conditions, such as type 2 diabetes or heart disease. This is partly due to the fact that society still deems hot flushes, night sweats and irregular periods as 'women's problems' that are merely part and parcel of the menopause transition. This 'normalization' of symptoms, however, can make women feel obliged to soldier on without a firm diagnosis. If this is you, now is not the time to keep calm and carry on…it's time to go and see your lovely doctor!

That being said, I do appreciate that some people need to pluck up the courage to make that initial appointment – for many, menopause is a very sensitive and personal issue – so here's my step-by-step guide to putting those wheels in motion and getting yourself checked out.

### Step 1: track your symptoms

If you think you may be perimenopausal (see pages 165–6), it's a really good idea to start tracking your symptoms. Try to do this for at least a month, up to a maximum of three months (by which time you'll have hopefully booked an appointment with your doctor).

By downloading a specialist menopause app (see Resources from page 241), you'll be able to track your symptoms and monitor any changes. From a clinical perspective, I really appreciate the fact that many menopause apps allow you to download your tracking data and take it along to your appointment. Analysing the timing, frequency and intensity of your symptoms can enable us to make a swift and accurate diagnosis.

If you're not app-minded, you can cross-reference your physical and psychological symptoms by reading this book, of course – head straight to pages 165–6 – or by accessing the NHS website. You can then jot down your observations in a diary, perhaps monitoring the timing and intensity of your hot flushes, or the regularity of your periods; anything, in fact, that you feel may be related to your fluctuating hormones.

All women in the UK are entitled to perimenopause/ menopause care on the NHS and should NOT have to use private healthcare.

## Step 2: prepare for your appointment

The more preparation you can do in advance, the better use you'll make of the time with your doctor. First and foremost, research your perimenopausal treatment options. If a patient arrives at my clinic with some basic knowledge of what's available to them, I might not need to start from scratch, and will therefore be able to spend more time discussing specifics and suitability.

You're essentially helping to direct your own consultation which, from my perspective, is always most welcome; it's a meeting of minds rather than a one-way process. You don't have to be a women's health expert, of course – leave that bit up to us! – but, as the old adage goes, information is power. By perusing this book, using an app, or browsing the NHS website, you'll be giving yourself a great head start.

From my experience, your first menopause-related appointment will involve general information gathering (you may not always receive hormonal or non-hormonal treatment at your initial consultation; this will often take place at the follow-up). Your doctor may also decide to check for any symptom overlap with other conditions, illnesses and deficiencies. Things like memory fog, hot flushes, anxiety attacks and low libido aren't always menopause-related, and can sometimes be attributed to other illnesses. Memory fog can be experienced by a patient with long Covid, for example, anxiety attacks can be caused by substance abuse, and hot flushes can sometimes indicate hyperthyroidism. As healthcare professionals, it's vital we think broadly.

Taking certain information to your appointment can be really helpful, too, not only to help us save time, but also to help us build a complete picture of you. You might consider gathering together the following:

- A list of symptoms (tracked via your menopause app, noted in your diary, or obtained from a Greene Climacteric Scale questionnaire, see Resources).
- Brief details of your immediate family's health history (such as diabetes, heart disease or cancer).
- A list of any prescribed or complementary medications you may be taking.
- Details of any allergies or intolerances you are prone to.
- A list of measures you are already trying (such as changing diet, stopping smoking).
- A blood pressure reading, if you have a monitor at home.
- Your latest height and weight measurements.

Some clinics will allow you to email the above information to your doctor in advance of your appointment; double-check this is the case by contacting the admin team or accessing the surgery's website. Mark your email for your doctor's attention, and it'll be forwarded to them prior to your consultation.

## Step 3: find out what you're entitled to

It's your body, it's your menopause, so it's only right you take control! Make yourself aware of what care you're entitled to and, when you make your appointment, don't be afraid to state your preferences.

- You can ask to be seen by a doctor who specializes in women's/menopausal health (most surgeries have at least one nowadays) – this may mean a longer wait for an appointment, however.
- If you feel uncomfortable being seen by a male doctor, ask the receptionist for an appointment with a female doctor.

- Bring a friend or relative with you to your appointment or put in an advance request for the surgery to provide a chaperone; this can be another health professional.
- You can request a double appointment in advance for your first perimenopause-related consultation, but availability will depend on your individual surgery policies.
- You should have the option of a face-to-face, telephone or video consultation (although I'd recommend that your first perimenopause-related appointment is in-person).
- If English isn't your first language, ask the receptionist to book a translator for you or bring someone along to interpret for you.

## Step 4: be proactive at your appointment!

As family doctors, we are committed to a person-centred approach, which means prioritizing the care and treatment that matters most to our patients, without judgement or assumption. For this reason, please don't be afraid to be upfront with your doctor when you see them; no one knows your body better than you, after all. The ideal appointment is a two-way process in which a doctor allows a patient to have their say, listens to their concerns and discusses options. Some diagnoses take longer to work out than others, but once you join up the dots and successfully prescribe the right treatment, both parties can experience a wonderful *eureka* moment.

It can be dispiriting for a patient to feel they're being fobbed off – I'm not a fan of that term, but I know it happens – or not taken seriously. Judging by some messages I receive on social media, this happens far too often. But rest assured, it is much less likely to happen if you follow steps 1, 2 and 3!

Asking your doctor the right questions can sometimes feel tricky, especially when appointment time is limited, but here are some common examples (all are subject to individual experiences, of course):

'I think I'm experiencing symptoms of perimenopause, such as... [then list your symptoms]. I've researched the hormonal and non-hormonal treatment options and would like your advice.'

'My quality of life has deteriorated since I've been having [then list your symptoms]. I've tried herbal treatments but they've not worked, so I'd like to find out more about HRT. Can you tell me about the risks and benefits?'

'I'd like to take oestrogen through the skin as a patch or a gel and, because I still have a uterus, I'd prefer to use body-identical progesterone.'

'I'm under 45 years old, so may I have an FSH (follicle stimulating hormone) blood test to exclude other causes for my symptoms?'

'I understand the FSH blood test might be repeated after six weeks, so I'll be around to have that done. I also understand that the FSH alone doesn't diagnose me as being in the perimenopausal phase; my symptoms (excluding other causes) can lead to the diagnosis...'

'I'm over 45 years old, I'm still having/not having periods, so I don't need an FSH (follicle stimulating hormone) blood test to diagnose that I'm perimenopausal.'

'I think my low mood may be due to hormone fluctuations. I'd prefer not to be prescribed anti-depressants and would like to discuss other options. I understand that HRT is a first-line treatment for menopausal symptoms, including psychological ones.'

# Menopause in trans & non-binary people

We need to be aware that research and conversations around menopause are usually framed around the experiences of cisgender women. For most individuals, this phase in life occurs in response to decreasing ovarian function; however, transgender and non-binary people can also experience symptoms of menopause even if the root causes differ.

AFAB (assigned female at birth) trans and non-binary people may take oestrogen blockers and testosterone in order to masculinize. Masculinizing hormone therapy does not usually cause menopausal symptoms but some individuals may experience hot flushes, night sweats, mood swings, lack of concentration, fatigue and sleepiness. Although masculinizing hormone therapy may decrease the risk of breast cancer, those who haven't had a complete subcutaneous mastectomy still need to remain breast-aware.

AMAB (assigned male at birth) trans and non-binary people may experience menopause-like symptoms (similar to those detailed above) if they are taking oestrogen-based hormonal treatment, which is often initiated before the age of 40.

Many of those in the trans and non-binary community receive little or no information about what to expect as they approach perimenopause and menopause. Moreover, there aren't enough fully trained specialists to help guide them through the process; as a consequence, a significant number of these patients do not get the care they need. Ideally, the management of their menopause symptoms – along with advice about NHS treatments available to them – should be overseen by a multidisciplinary team, which might incorporate the patient's doctor, a specialist in transgender health and a specialist in menopause care.

Positive steps are being taken to address this disparity, however, which I wholeheartedly welcome. In May 2022, the National Institute for Health and Care Excellence (NICE) announced plans to update its menopause guidance to include trans and non-binary individuals. This is encouraging news as it will undoubtedly benefit patients as well as professionals. For further guidance, see Resources from page 241.

Not all trans and non-binary people take hormones. A person can change their gender expression without any medical intervention.

# Breast cancer

Breast cancer is very common and, in the UK, about one in seven women will be diagnosed with it in their lifetime. Early detection significantly improves the chance of successful treatment and recovery, which is why it is so important to examine your breast tissue on a regular basis (see pages 16–17).

## Mammograms

Although younger women can get breast cancer, it affects more older people, and so anyone between the age of 50 and 71 who is registered with their doctor as a female and has breasts will be invited to have an NHS mammogram every three years. If you're 50 years old and have yet to be invited for a mammogram, it's perhaps worth speaking to your doctor. Another reason that mammograms are not routinely offered to younger women is that cancer cells appear white on a mammogram screening. Younger women have denser, oestrogen-rich breast cells, which also appear white on a mammogram. Therefore, it's harder to pick up white cancer cells on a white breast cell.

A mammogram is an X-ray screening of breast tissue that looks for cancerous growths that are often too small to see or feel. The X-ray machine usually takes an image from above and an image from the side of each breast.

If thanks to genetic testing or knowledge of your family history you know that you have a BRCA1, BRCA2 or TP53 genetic fault, or Lynch Syndrome (a genetic predisposition to certain cancers), you can have an early breast screening. Your doctor can help you access the screening programme best suited to you.

Trans men and non-binary people will receive an invite for a mammogram if they have breast tissue due to either naturally occurring oestrogen, or oestrogen hormone replacement. A trans man who's had a double mastectomy and male chest reconstruction will not usually have a screening, but will still need to remain vigilant. Sometimes a small amount of breast tissue can be left behind after the operation, and it's always a good idea to keep an eye out for lumps or any changes to the skin.

Patients usually receive results from a mammogram after about two weeks, via a letter that will be copied to your healthcare provider.

Typical outcomes would be:

♦ All clear with advice to self-examine (see pages 16–17) and if you are over 50 years, to have another mammogram in 3 years.

Self examination of the breasts is still of paramount importance!

◆ Unclear result with advice to have an ultrasound scan, an MRI and/or a fine-needle aspiration of a lump.

◆ Abnormal result with advice to see a breast cancer oncologist and a multidisciplinary team.

Anyone with an abnormal result will be referred for further tests and investigations (but this may not necessarily mean that cancer is present). Any treatment required will be handled by breast cancer specialists.

## Post-breast cancer care

Post-cancer care for those who have suffered breast cancer will vary for each individual. You will receive practical and emotional support from your oncologist, but may also benefit from the fabulous guidance offered by Breast Cancer Now specialist nurses, Macmillan nurses and Cancer Research UK (see Resources from page 241). They are so helpful and knowledgeable in all aspects of post-surgical care, and can offer advice about breast prostheses (artificial breast shapes), early menopause symptoms, sexual relationships, mental health support and financial/employment support. There is also a wealth of online information about breast health.

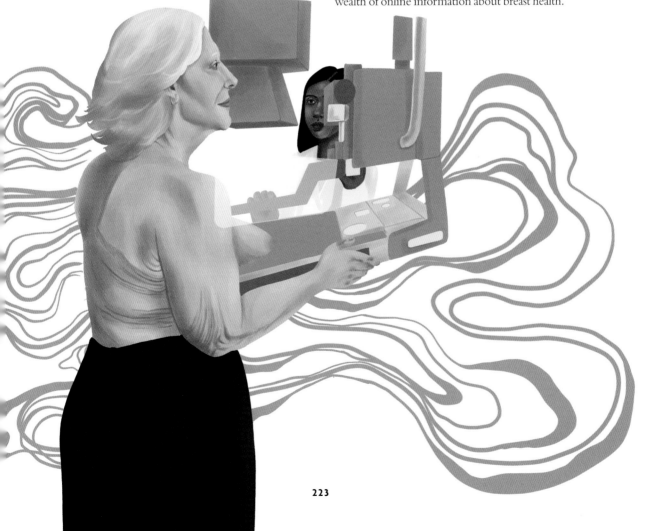

# Breast cancer in Black, Asian & ethnic minority communities

Genetic differences and structural racism within many systems of healthcare, public services and public information sadly mean that breast cancer is significantly more prevalent in some ethnicities than in others.

Black women are disproportionately affected by breast cancer; compared with white women, they have a 70 per cent higher chance of developing the disease and are more likely to lose their lives to it. There is no conclusive data on breast cancer in other ethnic minority communities, but, knowing what we know about the ethnicity gap in other areas of health, I believe this just shows the need for more research to be done!

'Triple-negative' types of cancer, which tend to be more aggressive and harder to treat, are much more common among Black women. The reasons for this can include the following:

* Black women having denser breast tissue, so it is more difficult to pick up cell changes on a mammogram.
* Less awareness of breast cancer in the community.
* Late presentation and lack of understanding of screening in ethnic minority communities.
* High rates of inflammatory breast cancer, an aggressive disease in which cancer cells block lymph vessels in the skin and develop changes in their DNA, giving the appearance of a red, swollen or inflamed breast.
* High rates of obesity.
* Barriers to healthcare linked to geographical areas of deprivation.
* Racism in the healthcare system.

Spotting the signs and symptoms of breast cancer isn't always straightforward among Black women. Skin colour makes certain changes to the breast harder to detect – like redness and dimpling, for instance – so be particularly vigilant during self examinations (see pages 16–17). Medical professionals also need to be extremely aware of this when consulting Black, Asian and ethnic minority patients. Do flag this with your doctor if you feel concerned and please attend your mammograms when called for them.

Black women have a **70% higher chance** of developing inflammatory breast cancer than white women

**Whatever your race or ethnicity, please attend your breast cancer screening when you are invited at the age of 50.**

# Dr Nighat's Takeaways

# 1 Keep a menopause symptom diary, using an app or a notebook

It's so useful for both you and your doctor!

# 2 Never deny yourself treatment

There are risks and benefits to every medication and if you put up barriers, your health and wellbeing might suffer.

# 3 Don't suffer in silence

Visit your doctor and ask questions. If there's something you don't know, ASK. There's no such thing as a daft question!

# 4 Your lifestyle underpins all health conditions

Maintaining a good diet, taking exercise, reducing alcohol intake, stopping smoking and recreational drug use, relieving stress and investing in self-care is vitally important.

# 5 Share your experience

Share your experience within your community, your workplace, your family and your friendship group. Your lived experience increases awareness, drives change, prompts research, reduces stigma and fights taboos.

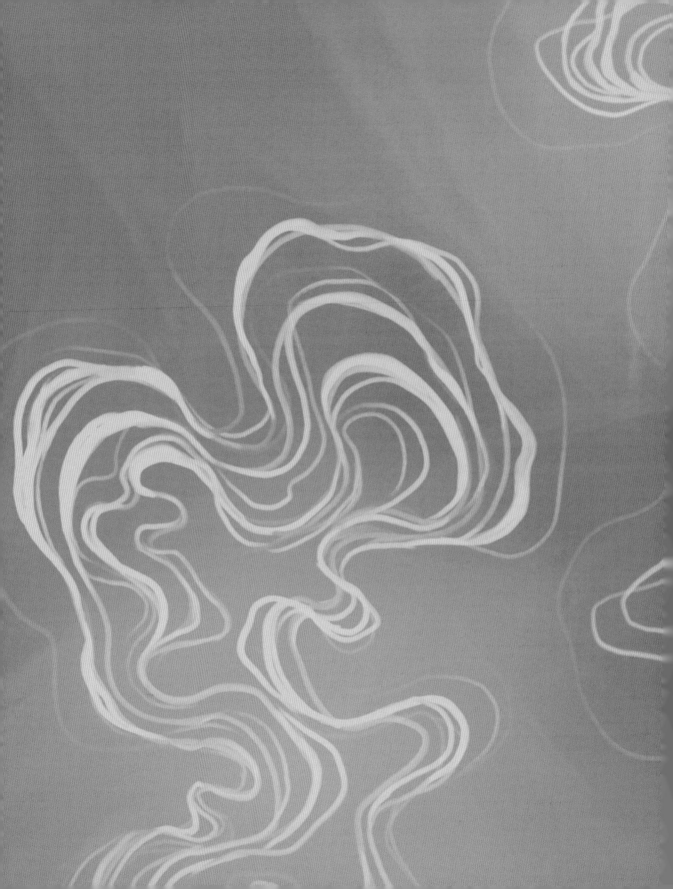

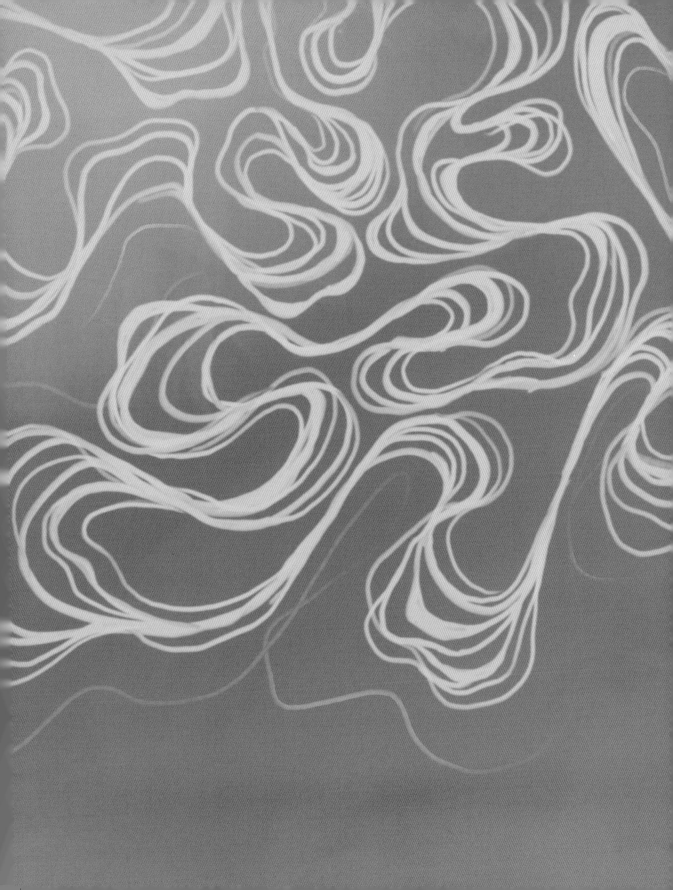

# Sharing the knowledge

There ends your journey of the three phases through which we all naturally progress: from starting our menstrual cycle, to working out our body through the fertility years, introducing new life into the world, and then the joy of our body then transitioning through to midlife.

Throughout our lives we need to be able to keep checking and understanding our bodies. Know what is normal for you. Understand when something is not right and know when to go to your doctor to show your concern.

I want to emphasize that the stigma and taboo around women's health and women's biology ends with this book. Enough with the lack of diversity and inclusion in medical textbooks. Enough with misrepresentation of neurodiverse women and those who are differently abled. Enough of ignoring ethnic minority communities. Enough of undermining and gaslighting women's bodies and their symptoms. Enough with not providing adequate pain relief for smear tests, childbirth and hysteroscopies. Enough of not showing real-life body shapes. Enough of lack of data. Enough of medical misogyny, which is perpetrated by the patriarchy – including the patriarchy within us and our own misgivings about whether our pain is worth discussing.

Hopefully by now you've recognized that I have absolutely no qualms talking about breasts, vulvas, vaginas, anuses – the lot! I think it's so important for women to be queens of their bodies, and as queens we should be fixing each other's crowns along the way.

This book is not mine; it is my gift to you. Take the knowledge within this book and share it like confetti with those around you.

*Nighat Arif*

Dr Nighat Arif

This book is my gift to you: take it, look after it, come back to it when you're ready, and know that you have the freedom to choose the care that suits you.

# GLOSSARY

**Abdomen** The region of the body between the chest and the pelvis that contains the digestive and reproductive (or abdominal) organs, often referred to as the belly.

**Abortion** The termination of a pregnancy before term; this can be medically induced or spontaneous (known as miscarriage).

**Adenoma** A non-cancerous cyst or tumour resembling glandular tissue arising from the layer of cells inside organs (epithelium).

**Adenomyosis** A condition in which the cells that normally line the uterine walls (endometrium) develop in the muscular wall of the uterus tissue, but continue to thicken and shed as part of the menstrual cycle. Unlike endometriosis, these cells are always inside the uterus.

**Amniotic fluid** The clear, watery fluid that surrounds a foetus in the uterus, cushioning it as the mother moves around and allowing the foetus to move freely.

**Amniotic sac** The membranous 'bag' surrounding a foetus in the uterus, which is filled with amniotic fluid.

**Anaemia** A condition in which the concentration of the oxygen-carrying pigment (haemoglobin) in red blood cells is too low. It can result because there are insufficient red blood cells or because those that are circulating are defective. It is not a disease, but a feature of different disorders.

**Anaesthetic** Literally means loss of sensation. In medicine, anaesthetics are used to numb sensation in certain areas (local anaesthetic), or to induce sleep for example for surgery (general anaesthestic).

**Anal sex** A form or sex in which a man's penis enters the anal passage of his partner.

**Androgen** Hormone that promotes the development and maintenance of male characteristics.

**Antenatal** Literally the time before birth of a baby. The term is mostly used to describe the care a mother receives during pregnancy prior to the birth.

**Antibiotic drugs** A group of drugs used to treat bacterial infections. They are sometimes offered to prevent infection if the immune system is impaired.

**Bacteria (single = bacterium)** Single-celled organisms abundant in air, soil and water, that are mostly harmless to humans. Some, such as gut bacteria, are beneficial and help break down food. A few, so-called pathogens, can cause disease.

**Barrier method of contraception** Forms of birth control, such as a condom or cap that physically prevent a sperm reaching an egg.

**Benign** A growth or tumour that is not cancerous. It may continue to grow in situ, but it will not spread to other parts of the body.

**Bilateral salpingo oophorectomy** Surgical procedure in which the ovaries and fallopian tubes are removed, often carried out as keyhole surgery.

**Bi-manual examination** A form of examination used to check internal organs in which the practitioner places one hand on the lower part of the person's abdomen and at the same time inserts two fingers into their vagina.

**Biopsy** A diagnostic test in which a small amount of tissue or a few cells are removed from the body for microscopic examination.

**Birth control** Any means of controlling fertility to prevent pregnancy, commonly described as contraception.

**Bloating** A feeling of fullness or swelling in the abdomen, possibly as a result of gas in the intestines, overeating, food intolerances or constipation.

**Blood clot** A mass of blood that forms if blood platelets, proteins and cells stick together. It can be carried around the body in the bloodstream or can become attached to wall of a blood vessel (thrombus).

**Body mass index (BMI)** A means of assessing whether a person is a healthy weight by measuring both weight and height – weight in kg/lbs is divided by height in metres/feet squared – then plotting the calculation on a chart, which gives a number, for example anything between 18.5–24.9 is a healthy weight, above 25 is overweight and above 30 is obese.

**Caesarean section/delivery** Also called a C-section, this is an operation to deliver a baby through an incision in the abdomen. It is usually performed if a vaginal delivery is medically risky or because a birth becomes difficult (emergency Caesarean).

**Cardiovascular disease** Disorders and diseases that affect the heart and blood vessels.

**Cervical mucus** The slippery discharge secreted by the cervix that makes it easier for sperm to swim up the vagina; its consistency changes during the menstrual cycle.

**Cervical screening** A regular screening test offered every 3–5 years in women aged 25 –65 that assesses the health of the cervix. Cells are taken from the cervix to check for types of human papillomavirus (HPV) that can cause cancerous changes.

**Cervix** The opening in the lower end of the uterus that leads to the vagina.

**Chaperone** A person who accompanies another, for example to a medical appointment.

**Cisgender (cis)** A person whose gender identity is the same as that identified at birth.

**Clitoris** Part of the female genitalia, this is a small sensitive erectile organ located just below the pubic bone, partly enclosed by the labia.

**Clot** *see* blood clot

**Coeliac disease** A condition in which the small intestine is hypersensitive to gluten, the protein found in wheat, rye and barley. Eating gluten causes the immune system to attack and damage the gut tissues, and as a result the person cannot absorb nutrients.

**Cognitive function** Term used to describe mental processes involved with the acquisition of knowledge, processing information and reasoning.

**Coil** A small T-shaped device inserted in the uterus to prevent pregnancy. There are two types: a copper coil (intrauterine device or IUD) and a hormone-releasing coil (intrauterine system or IUS).

**Combined oral contraceptive pill** Contraception in the form of a pill that contains artificial versions of the naturally occurring hormones progesterone and oestrogen.

**Conception** The beginning of pregnancy marked by the fertilization of an egg (ovum) by a sperm.

**Condom** A sheath-shaped barrier device used to prevent pregnancy and prevent sexually transmitted infections. Condoms can be placed over the penis or female versions (femidoms) are inserted into the vagina.

**Contraception** A means of controlling fertility to prevent pregnancy with barrier methods, coils or hormones.

**Contraceptive injection** An injection that releases the hormone progesterone into the bloodstream for longer-term pregnancy prevention; the effects can last between 8 and 13 weeks depending on the type.

**Contraceptive implant** Long-term form of contraception in which a small, flexible plastic rod is placed under the skin.

**Contractions, uterine** Rhythmic spasms of the muscles in the walls of the uterus that occur during childbirth.

**Copper coil** A small T-shaped implement inserted into the uterus as a form of contraception. This can be fitted at any point in the menstrual cycle.

**Corpus luteum** A cyst, or cluster of cells, which develops in the ovary during every menstrual cycle, just after an egg (ovum) leaves the ovary.

**Crabs** *see* Pubic lice

**Cramps, period** Known as dysmenorrhea, cramps are painful sensations that can occur when the body releases the hormone-like substances called prostaglandins that cause the uterus contract to expel its lining before and during a menstrual period.

**Cyclical HRT** A form of hormone replacement therapy (HRT) offered to women who have menopausal symptoms but who also still have their periods.

**Depression** A mood disorder that results in persistent feelings of sadness and hopelessness. Symptoms vary depending on the severity.

**Diabetes** A long-term metabolic disease characterized by high levels of blood sugar (glucose) in the body. Blood sugar is usually broken down by the hormone insulin. Diabetes can develop because the body produces no insulin (Type 1) or because the body cannot use the insulin it produces (Type 2) – the latter is often reversible.

**Gestational diabetes** A form of diabetes that can develop in pregnancy; this often resolves after pregnancy.

**Diagnosis** The process of identifying the nature of an illness by examination and assessment of the symptoms.

**Diaphragm** A barrier method of contraception that is fitted into the vagina to cover the cervix before vaginal sex.

**Discharge** Fluid that comes out of the body.

**Early menopause** This is the onset of menopause before the age of 40, and is also known as premature menopause or premature ovarian insufficiency (POI).

**Egg** A mature female reproductive cell (ovum) released from an ovary that, if fertilized, can develop into an embryo.

**Ejaculation** The action of ejecting semen from a male's body.

**Embryo** Human offspring in the process of development from fertilized egg to a foetus.

**Emergency contraception** This is contraception that can be given after unprotected sex to prevent a pregnancy. There are two forms: a person can take the morning-after pill, or a coil can be inserted.

**Endometrium** The inner lining of the uterus.

**Episiotomy** A surgical cut that can be made at the entrance of the vagina to help a difficult birth and prevent perineum tearing.

**Fallopian tube** One of two tubes that extend from the top of the uterus toward the ovaries, in which fertilization takes place. The ovum moves along the tube towards the main body of the uterus and the sperm travels from uterus towards the tube.

**Family planning**, *see* contraception

**Fasting cholesterol test** A blood test to check for cholesterol levels, for which the person is normally asked not to eat for 12 hours beforehand.

**Fertility** A person or couple's ability to produce offspring, which is dependent on age and health.

**Fertilization** The point at which a sperm enters an egg (ovum).

**Fibroid** A benign, slow-growing tumour formed of smooth muscle and connective tissue that can develop in the uterus. There can be one or more and the size can vary.

**Follicle** A small cavity in the body, for example a hair follicle. In an ovary, follicles are small sac-like, fluid-filled pouches, each of which contains one ovum (egg).

**GP** A general practitioner, or family doctor, is a doctor who assesses and treats common medical conditions, and refers patients to other medical disciplines for more specialist treatment when necessary.

**Gender** The sex that a person identifies themselves as, such as male, female or non-binary.

**Gender affirmation therapy** Any of several therapies, psychological and physical, that are offered to a person to help them live in their preferred gender identity.

**Gender diverse** A place that accommodates people of different genders, also an umbrella term used to address the spectrum of different gender identities.

**Genitals** A person's external sex organs.

**Gestation** The period of time between conception and birth during which an infant develops in the uterus, normally 40 weeks or 9 months .

**Gynaecological cancer** A cancer that affects any part of the reproductive system of a female.

**Gynaecologist** Doctor or surgeon specializing in the branch of medicine that focuses on female health and the female reproductive system.

**Hormone** Chemical messengers released into the bloodstream by certain organs that have a specific effect on tissues somewhere else in the body.

**Hot flush** A common symptom of the menopause, caused by hormonal imbalances, in which a person experiences a sudden rise in body temperature especially in the upper body, often accompanied by sweating, and looks flushed.

**Hyperthyroidism** Also known as overactive thyroid, a condition that results in overproduction of thyroid hormones. Symptoms include increase in heart rate, appetite and sweating, as well as weight loss.

**Hypothyroidism** Also known as underactive thyroid, a condition that results in inadequate levels of thyroid hormones, causing tiredness, lethargy and weight gain.

**Hysterectomy** The surgical removal of the uterus. The most common type involves only the uterus and cervix; sometimes the ovaries and fallopian tubes are also removed.

**Implantation** The point at which a fertilized egg (ovum) attaches itself to the wall of the uterus – this normally happens six days after fertilization.

**Incontinence** The involuntary passing of urine, which can be caused by injury, weakness or disease of the urinary tract.

**Infertility** Inability to produce a baby. This can be a result of a problem in the male or female reproductive systems, or both.

**Inflammation** Pain, swelling, heat and redness in one or several areas of the body as a result of an injury or infection.

**Insomnia** The inability to fall asleep or to stay asleep for any length of time. Causes can be physical, psychological or environmental.

**Insulin** The hormone produced by the pancreas that controls blood sugar levels in the body.

**Insulin resistance** A condition in which the body's cells do not respond properly to insulin whether it's produced by the body, or injected (in those with diabetes).

**Intercourse** Also known as sexual intercourse, this is physical contact between two individuals that involves genitalia of at least one of them.

**Intra-uterine device (IUD)** Small 'T'-shaped, non-hormonal device (coil) that is inserted into the uterus as a form of contraception.

**Intra-uterine system (IUS)** Small 'T'-shaped, hormone-releasing device (coil) that is inserted into the uterus as a form of contraception.

**Keloid scars** A scar that continues growing after a wound is healed and can grow to bigger than the original wound.

**LGBTQ+** Acronym used to refer to the group of people who identify as lesbian, gay, bisexual, transgender, queer or questioning. The '+' acknowledges that there are other sexual identities, such as intersex and asexual.

**Labia majora** The outer lips of the female external genitals.

**Labia minora** The inner lips of the female external genitals.

**Labour** The process by which an infant is born.

**Laparoscopy** A surgical procedure in which the interior of the abdomen is examined using a device called a laparoscope, which is inserted through a small hole ('key' hole) made in the abdominal wall.

**Libido** Level of sexual desire.

**Lubricant** An oily or slippery substance that can for example be used to reduce friction during intercourse.

**MRI scan** Short for magnetic resonance imaging, this is a diagnostic technique that produces a cross-sectional or three-dimensional images of organs or body structures.

**Mammogram** A type of X-ray used specifically to examine the breast for signs of cancer, offered as a form of screening.

**Mastectomy** Surgical removal of one or both breasts, usually to treat breast cancer.

**Menopause** The point in a woman's life when menstruation has ceased for 12 months, regardless of other symptoms.

**Menstruation** The periodic shedding of the lining of a woman's uterus that occurs if they are not pregnant.

**Midwife** A person trained to assist women in childbirth.

**Migraine** A type of headache characterized by recurrent attacks of severe pain, usually on one side of the head, which can cause throbbing sensation.

**Mini-pill** Also known as the progesterone-only pill (POP), this is a contraceptive pill that contains only progesterone, which works by thickening the cervical mucus and preventing the sperm reaching the egg.

**Miscarriage** The loss of a foetus before week 24 of pregnancy.

**Morning-after pill**, *see* Emergency contraception

**Multidisciplinary team** Healthcare team that is comprised of a number of different specialties, who work together to assist with a person's medical care.

**Myometrium** The muscle tissue in the wall of the uterus.

**Nausea** Feeling sick or the need to vomit.

**Needlestick injury** Accidental puncture of the skin by a potentially contaminated hypodermic needle, which carries a risk of disease.

**Neuropathic or neuropathy** Disease or inflammation affecting the peripheral nerves, the nerves that connect to the central nervous system (brain and spinal cord).

**NHS** The UK's health system – the National Health Service – which includes all healthcare practitioners.

**Non-binary** A person who does not identify themselves as either male or female.

**Obesity** A state of being very overweight; a person with a BMI above 30 is described as obese.

**Obstetrician** A doctor or surgeon specializing in the branch of medicine concerned with childbirth.

**Oestrogen(s)** A group of hormones essential for the maintenance of female characteristics of the body.

**Oestrogen-receptor-positive breast cancer (ER+)** A type of breast cancer with cells that have receptors that allow them to use oestrogen hormones to grow – so a person can be given medication to reduce the hormone production as a form of treatment.

**Off licence** Use of a drug or other preparation in a way that is not typically recommended by the manufacturer, but that is still safe.

**Oophorectomy** Surgical procedure in which the ovaries are removed.

**Oral medication** Medicines or tablets that are taken by mouth.

**Oral sex** Sexual activity in which one person's genitals are stimulated by the mouth of another person.

**Osteoporosis** Loss of bone tissue that causes bones to become brittle/fragile so are more likely to fracture. This is a natural part of aging, but women lose bone tissue faster after the menopause.

**Ovarian cyst** Abnormal, fluid-filled swelling that can develop on an ovary.

**Ovary** One of two glands, positioned either side of the uterus, in which eggs (ova) form and the female hormones oestrogen and progesterone are made.

**Ovulation** The process of the ovary releasing an egg (ovum).

**Ovum (plural = ova)** The mature female reproductive cell released from an ovary that, if fertilized, can develop into an embryo.

**Patch** An adhesive-plaster-like device that releases medication, for example for HRT or contraception, into the body through the skin; patch is normally changed every 2–3 weeks.

**Pelvis** Large bony, basin-like frame at the base of the spine that surrounds and protects the reproductive organs.

**Penetration** Physical contact between two individuals in which a man puts his penis into the vagina or anus of their partner.

**Penis** The largest external male sex organ.

**Perimenopause** The time before the menopause when a woman has symptoms of the menopause, but is still menstruating; this can last up to a decade.

**Perinatal phase** The weeks immediately before and after the birth of a baby.

**Perineum** The part of the body between the entrance to the vagina (or the scrotum) and the anus.

**Period** Also known as menstruation, this is the periodic shedding of the lining of a woman's uterus that occurs if they are not pregnant.

**Pessary** Medical device placed into the vagina, for example, to correct the position of the uterus or to deliver medication or contraception.

**Physiotherapist** Healthcare professional who provides physical therapy treatment to help prevent or reduce joint stiffness and aid movement.

**Pituitary gland** Situated under the brain, this is the most important gland of the endocrine (hormone-producing) system. Called the master gland, it controls and regulates all the other endocrine glands and many body processes.

**Placenta** The organ formed in the uterus during pregnancy that supports and nourishes the foetus.

**Placental abruption** Separation of the placenta from the wall of the uterus during pregnancy or labour before the baby is born; this is life-threatening to mother and baby.

**Polyp** A growth, often from a stalk, that projects from the wall of an organ, such as the cervix, uterus, or nose. Some are cancerous and need to be removed.

**Post-menopause** The life stage of a woman, or person assigned a woman at birth, after the menopause.

**Post-natal** The first weeks after the birth of a baby.

**Post-partum** The hours immediately after the birth of a baby.

**Premature menopause** Menopause that begins when a woman is under the age of 40 years.

**Progesterone** Hormone made in the ovaries that is essential to the functioning of the female reproductive system.

**Progesterone-only pill (POP)** *see* Mini pill

**Progestogen drugs** A group of drugs containing properties similar to naturally occurring hormone progesterone that are used in contraceptives.

**Prolapse** Displacement of an organ, for example the uterus, from its normal place in the body.

**Puberty** The time during which a girl (or boy) becomes sexually mature.

**Pubic lice** Tiny parasitic insects, often called crabs, that can attach themselves to the skin and hair of the areas around the genital. Spread by close physical contact they cause intense itching; lice and/or eggs may be visible.

**Pulmonary embolism** Obstruction of one of the arterial blood vessels in the lungs by a blood clot. Clots can form in the lungs or be carried there from another part of the circulatory system by the blood.

**Screening** The regular testing of apparently healthy members of the population to check for signs of diseases.

**Semen** The sperm-containing fluid released from the penis during ejaculation/orgasm.

**Sequential HRT** A form of hormone replacement therapy for women who still menstruate that involves taking one hormone daily (oestrogen), then additional progesterone for part (normally half) of the month.

**Sexuality** A person's identity in relation to the genders they are attracted to, and/or how they identify their own sexuality. It also describes a person's attitude and behaviour towards sex and physical intimacy with others.

**Sexually transmitted diseases (STDs)** Diseases that are transmitted through sexual contact with another person.

**Side effect** The secondary response caused by a drug beyond the intended therapeutic effects.

**Smear test** Routine screening test offered every 3–5 years to all women (or those assigned female at birth) aged 25–65 in which cells are collected from the cervix to check for types of human papillomavirus (HPV) that can cause cancerous changes in the cervix.

**Speculum** Device placed in the vagina by a healthcare professional so that the cervix can be checked, and a smear test can be carried out.

**Sperm** The male sex cell that responsible for fertilization on an egg (ovum).

**Spotting** Light traces of blood that can indicate the end of a period, or that are sometimes seen around ovulation.

**Stress incontinence** Involuntary loss of urine that occurs, for example, when a person coughs or lifts a heavy object, because the muscles at the exit to the urinary tract (sphincter) are weakened, for example after childbirth.

**Surrogacy** The process of carrying and giving birth to a baby for another person. The birth mother then hands over custody of the baby to that person.

**Swab** Small absorbent pad or cloth (generally sterile) used in surgery or by healthcare professional to clean a wound, apply medication or take a specimen.

**Synthetic** A chemically made substance that imitates a naturally occurring product.

**Systemic** Medical treatment using substances/drugs that travel throughout the body.

**Testosterone** The hormone that stimulates the development of, and maintains, secondary male characteristics.

**Tinnitus** Continuous or intermittent ringing, buzzing or roaring sound in one, or more commonly both, ears.

**Topical** A medication or treatment applied directly to an area (of skin, for example).

**Toxic shock syndrome** A rare, but potentially life-threatening, condition caused by harmful bacteria getting into the body and releasing toxins. It is sometimes associated with tampon use in young women.

**Trans man** Person living as a man who was assigned female gender at birth.

**Trans woman** Person living as a woman who was assigned male gender at birth.

**Transdermal** Application of a drug through the skin, typically via an adhesive patch.

**Transgender, or trans** A person who is not living as the gender they were assigned at birth.

**Transvaginal ultrasound scan** An ultrasound scan carried out using a probe inserted into the vagina, *see* also Ultrasound scan

**Trimester** The three 'periods' of pregnancy, each covering around one-third of the pregnancy.

**Triple-negative cancer** An aggressive, fast-growing form of breast cancer in which the cells do not have hormone receptors that they use for growth.

**Ultrasound scan** A diagnostic tool in which high-frequency sound waves are passed through the body – the reflected echoes build a picture of the organs, or foetus for example, visible on a screen.

**Unprotected sex** Sexual intercourse with no form of contraception.

**Urethra** The opening, or sphincter, at the end of the ureter through which urine flows out of the body.

**Urge incontinence** The uncontrolled leakage of urine that occurs when a person feels a sudden urge to pee and is unable to stop the flow.

**Uterus** Largest internal female reproductive organ in which a foetus remains during pregnancy.

**Vaccine** A medical preparation that is given to induce immunity to an infectious disease. Some require several doses to take effect and for others one dose provides life immunity.

**Vagina** The muscular tube, or canal, between the external female genitalia (vulva) and the internal organs of the cervix and the uterus.

**Vaginal mucus** Slimy substance secreted by the vagina that varies in consistency.

**Vaginal oestrogen** A form of oestrogen (female hormone) that is administered in the form or a pessary or cream into the vagina.

**Virus** Simple, small microorganisms that replicate inside cells and can cause disease.

**Vulva** The external female genitals.

**Withdrawal method** A method to avoid pregnancy when the penis is removed from the vagina before orgasm/ejaculation to prevent sperm entering the vagina.

**Womb** The non-medical word used to describe uterus.

**X-ray** A diagnostic tool that involves passing electromagnetic radiation of short wavelength and high energy through the body to view bones, organs and internal tissues.

# RESOURCES

## FAIR HEALTHCARE ACCESS FOR ALL

**Women's health & disability**

Sisters of Frida organization, a collective of disabled women: www.sisofrida.org

**Trans patient training for doctors**

GPs can access an excellent module on the Royal College of GP's LGBT Health Hub: www.elearning.rcgp.org.uk

The Gender GP online clinic also contains a wealth of useful information for physicians and patients: www.gendergp.com

## PHASE 1: YOUR PUBERTY YEARS

**Periods**

Wellbeing of Women charity: www.wellbeingofwomen.org.uk

**Period tracking apps**

Flo: www.flo.health

Clue: www.helloclue.com

Ovia Health: www.oviahealth.com

**Period inequality**

Plan International: www.plan-international.org

The Trussell Trust: www.trusselltrust.org

Binti International: www.bintiperiod.org

**Premenstrual dysphoric disorder**

International Association for Premenstrual Disorders (IAPMD) self-screening test: www.iapmd.org/self-screen

**Violence against women & girls**

Childline: www.childline.org.uk; Helpline: 0800 1111

Women's Aid: www.womensaid.org.uk

SWGfL, a charity offering support for online abuse: www.swgfl.org.uk

Karma Nirvana, working to end honour-based abuse: www.karmanirvana.org.uk

**Female genital mutilation**

FGM-related help, advice and support is available from a number of charitable organizations.

Action Aid: www.actionaid.org.uk

Oxfam: www.oxfam.org

UN Women: www.unwomen.org

Women & Girls Network: www.wgn.org.uk

**Contraception & sexual health**

Brook, offering confidential advice for young people: www.brook.org.uk

Health for Teens: www.healthforteens.co.uk

NHS advice and information: www.letstalkaboutit.nhs.uk

**Sexually transmitted diseases**

The following websites contain some really useful information:

Brook, offering confidential advice for young people: www.brook.org.uk

Better2Know, offering sexual health testing services: www.better2know.co.uk

Terrence Higgins Trust, an HIV and sexual health charity: www.tht.org.uk

**Gender identity**

The following resources contain some useful information:

Gender Identity Development Service: www.gids.nhs.uk

Trans Actual: www.transactual.org.uk

Welsh Gender Service: www.cavuhb.nhs.wales/our-services/welsh-gender-service

National Gender Identity Clinical Network for Scotland: www.ngicns.scot.nhs.uk/gender-identity-clinics

Regional Gender Identity Service for Northern Ireland: www.belfasttrust.hscni.net/service/regional-gender-identity-service/

Regional Gender Identity Clinic for Northern Ireland (under-18s): www.familysupportni.gov.uk/Search/Details/5033?slug=gender-identity-clinic--camhs-belfast

### Egg preservation for trans people

Human Fertilisation & Embryology Authority (HFEA): www.hfea.gov.uk

### Mental health & trans people

Stonewall, a UK-based charity that stands for the freedom, equity and potential of all lesbian, gay, bi, trans, queer, questioning and ace (LGBTQ+) people: www.stonewall.org.uk

### Young people visiting a GP alone

NSPCC, offering advice about the Gillick competence and Fraser guidelines: https://learning.nspcc.org.uk/child-protection-system/gillick-competence-fraser-guidelines

# PHASE 2: YOUR FERTILITY YEARS

### Pregnancy & childbirth

General advice and guidance can be found on these websites:

Tommy's, a pregnancy charity: www.tommys.org

Emma's Diary: www.emmasdiary.co.uk

National Childbirth Trust: www.nct.org.uk/pregnancy

NHS pregnancy advice: www.nhs.uk/pregnancy

### Second & third pregnancy trimesters

The following books offer good advice:

*The Modern Midwife's Guide to Pregnancy, Birth and Beyond* by Marie Louise

*Hypnobirthing: Practical Ways to Make Your Birth Better* by Siobhan Miller

*What to Expect When You're Expecting* by Heidi Murkoff

*Pregnancy for Men: The Whole Nine Months* by Mark Woods

*The Expectant Dad's Survival Guide* by Rob Kemp

### Having a baby if you're LGBT+

NHS advice: www.nhs.uk/pregnancy/having-a-baby-if-you-are-lgbt-plus/

### Help with quitting smoking

NHS advice and app: www.nhs.uk/better-health/quit-smoking/

### Health & fitness resources

NHS BMI calculator: www.nhs.uk/live-well/healthy-weight/bmi-calculator

NHS healthy eating guidance: www.nhs.uk/live-well/eat-well/

NHS Couch to 5K: www.nhs.uk/live-well/exercise/running-and-aerobic-exercises/get-running-with-couch-to-5k

My Fitness Pal: www.myfitnesspal.com

Lose It! weight loss plan: www.loseit.com

### Eating disorders

BEAT, a charity offering great practical support: www.beateatingdisorders.org.uk

National Centre for Eating Disorders: www.eating-disorders.org.uk

### Unplanned pregnancies & ending a pregnancy

Brook, offering confidential advice for young people: www.brook.org.uk

British Pregnancy Advisory Service: www.bpas.org.uk

Pregnancy Crisis Helpline: www.pregnancycrisishelpline.org.uk; Helpline: 0800 368 9296

National Unplanned Pregnancy Advice Service: www.nupas.co.uk

Marie Stopes Clinics for abortion care services: www.msichoices.org.uk

Planned Parenthood, a US-based organization for advice and guidance: www.plannedparenthood.org

### Miscarriage support

Tommy's, a pregnancy charity offering support for baby loss: www.tommys.org

Miscarriage Association for miscarriage support: www.miscarriageassociation.org.uk

Sands, support for stillbirth and neonatal loss: www.sands.org.uk

Lullaby Trust, offering emotional support for bereaved
families of Sudden Infant Death Syndrome:
www.lullabytrust.org.uk
*Life After Baby Loss* by Nicola Gaskin

**Premature birth**
Bliss, offering support for babies born premature or
sick: www.bliss.org.uk

**Ectopic pregnancy**
The Ectopic Pregnancy Trust has some really useful
information: www.ectopic.org.uk

**Pregnancy in Black & ethnic minority communities**
Maternal Mental Health Alliance:
www.maternalmentalhealthalliance.org
Black women's maternity experiences report:
www.fivexmore.com

**PCOS**
British and Irish Hypertension Society: www.bihsoc.org
Verity, a PCOS support charity based on Twitter:
@veritypcos
PCOS Awareness Association: www.pcosaa.org
PCOS Vitality: www.pcosvitality.com
DAISy-PCOS for PCOS research: www.daisypcos.com
Cysters: www.cysters.org

**Endometriosis**
Endometriosis UK has a fabulous website for
information: www.endometriosis-uk.org

**IVF**
ICB guidelines and NICE recommendations on NHS
in-vitro fertilization (IVF) availability:
www.nhs.uk/conditions/ivf/availability
The British Infertility Counselling Association provides
advice and guidance to people of all ages who are
considering fertility treatment and preservation:
www.bica.net
The Fertility Network UK campaigns for equitable
access to NHS-funded fertility treatment:
www.fertilitynetworkuk.org
Proud 2b Parents, for LGBTQ+ parents seeking IVF
advice: www.proud2bparents.co.uk
Stonewall, advice for LGBTQ+ parents:
www.stonewall.org.uk

**Mental health during pregnancy**
Mind: www.mind.org.uk
Tommy's, a pregnancy charity: www.tommys.org
Pandas, perinatal mental illness support:
www.pandasfoundation.org.uk

**Gynaecological cancer support**
Target Ovarian Cancer offers some great tools and
resources: www.targetovariancancer.org.uk
The Eve Appeal, a wonderful gynaecological cancer
charity: www.eveappeal.org.uk

**Breast health & post-cancer care**
Breast Cancer Now: www.breastcancernow.org
Macmillan Cancer Support: www.macmillan.org.uk
CoppaFeel, a breast cancer charity:
www.coppafeel.org.uk (also great on Twitter, TikTok
and Instagram)
Cancer Research UK: www.cancerresearchuk.org

# PHASE 3: YOUR MIDLIFE YEARS
**Premature menopause**
The Daisy Network offers advice and raises awareness
of POI: www.daisynetwork.org
For a deeper dive into these conditions, I thoroughly
recommend The Complete Guide to POI and
Early Menopause by Dr Hannah Short and Mandy
Leonhardt

**Testosterone**
To learn more about this hormone, watch Kate Muir's
fantastic documentary Davina McCall: Sex, Mind &
the Menopause (produced by Louise Perrie)
Menopause Mandate campaign group, working hard
to effect change in the way testosterone can be
prescribed: www.menopausemandate.com
Menopause Support: www.menopausesupport.co.uk

**Skin-safe vaginal moisturizers & lubricants**
Jo Divine: www.jodivine.com

**Risks of HRT**
National Institute for Health and Care Excellence, up-
to-the-minute guidelines: www.nice.org.uk
Balance menopause app with Dr Louise Newson:
www.balance-menopause.com/menopause-library/

putting-the-risks-of-taking-hrt-into-perspective-
with-sign-language

### Complementary therapies to control menopause symptoms

Complementary Medicine Association, a great
information bank for patients and fellow GPs: www.
the-cma.org.uk

Balance menopause app with Dr Louise Newson has a
section on complementary therapies: www.balance-
menopause.com

Acupuncture World Information Center, with
accredited acupuncture therapists:
www.acupuncture.org

The National Institute of Medical Herbalists, with a list
of accredited practitioners: www.nimh.org.uk

Every Mind Matters initiative, with more information
about cognitive behavioural therapy (CBT): www.
nhs.uk/every-mind-matters

Women's Health Concern, offering a really useful CBT
factsheet: www.womens-health-concern.org

### Healthy eating

Dr Mary Claire Haver, a US-based obstetrics and
gynaecology physician who specializes in women's
nutrition: @thegalvestondiet on Instagram

### Improving sleep

Sleepio, a handy sleep app: www.sleepio.com
Calm, another sleep app: www.calm.com

### Exercise

I often recommend the following exercise-related
resources to my patients:

NHS Couch to 5K: www.nhs.uk/live-well/exercise/
running-and-aerobic-exercises/get-running-with-
couch-to-5k

Her Spirit: www.herspirit.co.uk
This Girl Can: www.thisgirlcan.co.uk

### Perimenopause & metal health

*Perimenopausal Depression: An Under-Recognised
Entity* by Jayashri Kulkarni: www.ncbi.nlm.nih.gov/
pmc/articles/PMC6299176

NHS mental health advice; self-referral to NHS Talking
Therapies services: www.nhs.uk/mental-health

Mind, a charity offering help with mental health issues:
www.mind.org.uk

### Menopause in trans & non-binary people

Rock My Menopause, an inclusive and informative
resource offering guidance for trans and non-binary
people: www.rockmymenopause.com

Gender GP (UK-based): www.gendergp.com

National Center for Transgender Equality (US-based):
www.transequality.org

### Tracking menopause symptoms

NHS symptom lists (search for 'perimenopause' or
'menopause'): www.nhs.uk

Health and Her, offering a menopause tracking app:
www.healthandher.com

Stella menopause tracking app: www.onstella.com

Balance menopause app, my personal favourite, with
Dr Louise Newson, a fantastic little tool that not
only enables you to record and recognize your
symptoms, but also allows you to interact with an
online community of like-minded people: www.
balance-menopause.com

Greene Climacteric Scale (GCS) questionnaire: this
is widely available online, for example here: www.
ardblair.scot.nhs.uk/your-record/electronic-reviews/
menopause-symptom-scale-greene-climacteric/

### Urinary incontinence & bladder health

Bladder Health UK, a charity offering some
really helpful advice and information: www.
bladderhealthuk.org

## STATISTICS RESOURCES

**Page 27:** 8.9% of the residents of England and Wales did
not have English as their main language in 2021 (Office
for National Statistics 2021 Census, 29 November 2022.
www.ons.gov.uk/peoplepopulationandcommunity/
culturalidentity/language/bulletins/
languageenglandandwales/census2021)

**Page 43:** 13% of UK schoolgirls missed a day of
school every month due to their period ('Nearly two
million girls miss school because of their period',
Plan International website, 20 October 2021. www.
plan-uk.org/media-centre/nearly-two-million-

girls-in-the-uk-miss-school-because-of-their-period#:~:text=Nearly%20two%20million%20girls%20(64,children's%20charity%20Plan%20International%20UK)

**Page 52:** A year's worth of disposable period products contributes 5.3kg of C02 ('Which Period Products are Best for the Environment?', by Leah Rodriguez, Global Citizen website, 27 May 2021. www.globalcitizen.org/en/content/best-period-products-for-the-environment/)

**Page 54:** The average woman in the UK will spend up to £18,450 on products geared towards her period over a lifetime ('Women Spend More than £18,000 on Having Periods in Their Lifetime, Study Reveals', by Rachel Moss, The Huffington Post UK website, 3 September 2015. www.huffingtonpost.co.uk/2015/09/03/women-spend-thousands-on-periods-tampon-tax_n_8082526.html)

**Page 55:** A 2017 survey revealed that nearly half of daughters in the UK said they'd feel uncomfortable discussing periods with their fathers ('1 in 4 UK women don't understand their menstrual cycle', Action Aid website, 23 May 2017. https://www.actionaid.org.uk/blog/news/2017/05/24/1-in-4-uk-women-dont-understand-their-menstrual-cycle)

**Page 66:** Globally 29% of all women of reproductive age are affected by anaemia (The Global Prevalence of Anaemia in 2011 by World Health Organization, 2015. apps.who.int/iris/bitstream/handle/10665/177094/9789241564960_eng.pdf)

**Page 74:** 27% of couples practicing the withdrawal method will get pregnant each year ('Withdrawal as a pregnancy prevention associated risk factors among US high school students: findings from the 2011 National Youth Risk Behavior Study' by Nicole Liddon, Emily O'Malley Olsen, Marion Carter and Kendra Hatfield-Timajchy, Contraception: An international reproductive health journal, February 2016. www.contraceptionjournal.org/article/S0010-7824(15)00571-5/fulltext)

**Page 92:** 46% of trans people in the UK have experienced suicidal thoughts (LGBT in Britain Health Report, by Chaka L Bachmann (Stonewall) and Becca Gooch (YouGov), 7 November 2018. https://www.stonewall.org.uk/system/files/lgbt_in_britain_health.pdf)

**Page 105:** 1 in 7 couples in the UK are affected by infertility (NHS data, accessed 1 March 2023. www.nhs.uk/conditions/infertility)

**Page 110:** 1 in 6 adoptions in England in 2021 were to same-sex couples ('Children looked after in England including adoption: 2020 to 2021, Department for Education Gov.uk website, 18 November 2021. https://www.gov.uk/government/statistics/children-looked-after-in-england-including-adoption-2020-to-2021)

**Page 121:** Black women in the UK are 4 times more likely to die in pregnancy and childbirth than white women ('Saving Lives, Improving Mothers' Care: Lessons learned to inform maternity care from the UK and Ireland Confidential Enquiries into Maternal Deaths and Morbidity 2017–19', Mothers and Babies: Reducing Risk through Audits and Confidential Enquiries across the UK, November 2021. https://www.npeu.ox.ac.uk/assets/downloads/mbrrace-uk/reports/maternal-report-2021/MBRRACE-UK_Maternal_Report_2021_-_FINAL_-_WEB_VERSION.pdf)

**Page 141:** By age 35, 60% of Black women are thought to have uterine fibroids, compared to 6% of white women ('Understanding Racial Disparities for Women with Uterine Fibroids' by Beata Mostafavi, Michigan Medicine, University of Michigan website, 12 August 2020. https://www.michiganmedicine.org/health-lab/understanding-racial-disparities-women-uterine-fibroids#:~:text=Nearly%20a%20quarter%20of%20Black,fibroids%20or%20suffer%20from%20complications)

**Page 166:** 1 in 4 women said a lack of support for menopause symptoms in the workplace has left them unhappy in their job ('More than 1m UK women could quit their jobs through lack of menopause support' by Amelia Hill, the guardian website, 17 January 2022. https://www.theguardian.com/society/2022/jan/17/more-than-1m-uk-women-could-quit-their-jobs-through-lack-of-menopause-support)

**Page 182:** 81.9% of postmenopausal women have low levels of magnesium ('The Severity of Depressive Symptoms vs. Serum MG and Zn Levels in Postmenopausal Women', by M. Stanisławska,

M. Szkup-Jabłonska, A. Jurczak, S. Wieder-Huszla,
Samochowiec, Jasiewicz, I. Nocen, K. Augustyniuk, A.
Brodowska, B. Karakiewicz, D. Chlubek and E. Grochans,
Biological Trace Element Research 157, January 2014.
https://doi.org/10.1007/s12011-013-9866-6)

**Page 189:** over 1/3 of women who visited their
doctor with perimenopausal symptoms were
offered antidepressants ('Menopausal women
wrongly prescribed antidepressants which make
their symptoms worse, warn experts' by Maya
Oppenheim, the Independent website, 10 October
2019. https://www.independent.co.uk/news/health/
menopause-antidepressants-symptoms-worse-hrt-
shortage-a9148951.html)

**Page 215:** on average women of colour experience
perimenopause earlier than their white counterparts
and experience perimenopausal symptoms for a
longer period ('What Experts Want Women of Color
to Know about Menopause' by Beth Levine, Everyday
Health website, 13 January 2022. https://www.
everydayhealth.com/menopause/what-experts-want-
bipoc-women-to-know-about-menopause/)

**Page 224:** Black women have a 70% higher chance
of developing inflammatory breast cancer than
white women ('New Research Highlights Disparity in
Inflammatory Cancer Survival Rates', Rogel Cancer
Center University of Michigan Health website, 10
December 2020. https://www.rogelcancercenter.
org/news/archive/new-research-highlights-disparity-
inflammatory-cancer-survival-rates)

# INDEX

# ACKNOWLEDGEMENTS

This book and my medical career so far would not have been possible without the help and support of so many people. It's true that it really does take a village! And in particular I'd like to thank the following people and organisations.

I want to say a huge thank you to my family. My parents, whose duas (prayers) and guidance continues to support me, and my siblings, Irfan, Imran, Saba and Ali, who will always be my best friends. My husband, Khalid, is a pillar of support, a dad to our three boys, and a soundboard for the choices I make. To my children, Haris, Qasim and Adam, who are my world and provide so much fun in my life. To the Pakistani women in my community: when I first arrived in the UK, they provided so much food, love, education and embraced us with open arms. These incredible women continue to teach me the facets of womanhood to this day.

When it comes to medicine and women's health, I am fully aware that I stand on the shoulders of giants, in particular Dr Louise Newson, who gave me the courage to push my understanding on HRT and menopause care and translate that to my South Asian community. Dr Annice Mukherjee made me understand the impact of hormones in women, and to Dr Radikha Vohra , Dr Aziza Sesey, Dr Liz O'Riordan, Dr Philippa Kaye, Dr Zoe Williams, Dr Larissa, Dr Sara Hyat, Dr Punam Krishan, Dr Naomi Potter – whose book with Davina McCall I contributed to – thank you for your support.

Thank you also to my colleagues from the US from whom I learn so much: Dr Karen Tang, Dr Mary Claire Haver and Dr Rachel Rubin.

To all the people who have contributed towards getting this book into its current state, thank you. In particular, Dr Ajay Verma who has been immensely helpful in providing me with education and support when proofreading sections of the book, and Dr Kamilah Kamaruddin, who is a voice for trans rights in the medical community and gave her wise insight into the sections on healthcare for trans people.

A huge thank you to my family at Wellbeing of Women, especially Dame Lesley Regan, Janet Lindsay, who brought me on as an ambassador, and my fellow ambassador Rosie Nixon, for her constant support. Thanks also to Manjit Gill MBE from Binti Period, whose campaigning about periods is invaluable and who contributed her knowledge about the myths around menstrual cycles, and to Hibo Wardere and Nimko Ali OBE, whose advice helped me to write about FGM with clarity and authority. I'm eternally grateful for grassroots campaigners who do so much for women's health: Diane Danzebrink, founder of Menopause Support; Elizabeth Carr-Ellis From Pausitivity; and South Asian breast cancer campaigns and campaigners, Sakoon Through Cancer, Iyna Butt, Kreena Dhiman and Bep Dhaliwal. And thank you to the charities: The Eve Appeal, Jo's Cervical Cancer Trust, Breast Cancer Now, Lichen Sclerosus and Vulval

Cancer UK Awareness who have been a wealth of information and have always supported my work.

Thanks to Jan Croxson, my agent, who found me in 2019, met me for 30 seconds and said she'd like to sign me. I was gobsmacked that somebody would take a punt on a hijab-wearing, slightly potty-mouthed, Muslim woman with three kids and take me into the world of media along with Borra Garson and Louise Leftwich. To Davina McCall for being so supportive and lifter of women.

To Kate Muir who originally asked me to be involved with Davina McCall: Sex, Myths and the Menopause. To Eleanor Mills who helped me to write about women's health and who brought me on as an ambassador for Noon.

A huge thank you to the BBC Breakfast team: Louise Minchin for being a guide and mentor, Naga Munchetty, Sally Nugent, and Richard (or 'Freddie') who has been so supportive of my media work and has always requested to get me onto the show.

Thanks to the dream team at ITV's This Morning: Phil and Holly for being extremely supportive, Alison Hammond, Dermot O'Leary for always being so kind, as well as Editor Martin Frizell and Assistant Producer Ellie Cole, who are so supportive of having someone like me on screen on a weekly basis. And Josie Gibson, telling me I was her favorite doctor has been the icing on the cake (though I'm sure she says that to everybody!)

Thanks also to my BBC Three Counties Radio team, especially Louise Parry, and Toby Friedner, who tried to teach me the art of presenting on a Sunday morning when I've had little to no breakfast and half a cup of tea, but with whom it's been an absolute blast to learn – there is more to presenting than I was ever aware of.

Thank you Baroness Sayeeda Warsi, Saira Khan, Anita Rani, Pippa Vosper, Lavina Mehta MBE, Meera Bhogal, Tessy Ojo CBE, for always championing my work. My HerSpirit friends: Mel Berry, Holly Woodford and Professor Greg Whyte, who literally motivate me to do exercise and get fitter, stronger, healthier in every way because I consume more chocolate than I should!

A huge thank you to my NHS surgery, in particular my supportive colleagues Dr Heather White, Dr Kirsten Riemer and Dr Lee Mitchell. To all my colleagues at OSD Healthcare who helped me set up a private women's health clinic to my own exacting specifications, even getting Entonox for pain relief in my coil insertion clinics. And to my NHS patients, who through their lived experience, have been more of an education than any medical textbook.

A massive thank you to Stephanie Jackson for believing in the vision of this book and taking on this huge gauntlet of a project. I'm so grateful to Jo Lake and Han, whose wisdom and advice I very much appreciated. I'm also grateful to Pauline Bache, Jaz Bahra, and Liliana Rasmussen for all their help, without Liliana's illustrations, this book would not have the soul that it does have.

My teachers at the Misbourne School, in particular my head teacher David Selman, who refused to make me head-girl so I could concentrate on my A-levels and become the first student from the school to go on to study medicine, thank you. Mrs Carol Taylor who provided me with mentorship and tissues as I cried in her office on a practically daily basis for fear of failure (she always had shortbread biscuits and tea); Ms Lorraine Cummings who helped me do my UCAS application to get into Queen Mary's University of London Barts and the London School of Medicine. And to all the professors, friends, lecturers at Barts who put me on my journey to becoming a doctor.

Finally to nine-year-old me, the little Nighat, who was so lost and had left everything she had known in Pakistan. She was in an alien world, never having the right clothing for the wet and cold weather, not understanding the new food and way of life, but she also gained all these freedoms and was able to not be hindered as a girl. Moving here, I felt a bittersweet loss of my life in Pakistan but I also realized a love of what I found in the UK. There's no other place like my home town of Chesham. When I came here as that young girl I was constantly battling to try and find my identity, so I want to say thank you to that girl, because she persevered with a smile (still, when I'm nervous I smile, which is why I'm always smiling on TV!) and for gradually loosened the shackles of the patriarchy in a small way, being slightly rebellious and finding company in medicine. Because of that, this book is for all the other people who have a sense of loss of identity and loss of grounding – and who every now and then say to themselves, What am I doing? I hope that you can at least feel like you have a handle on and an understanding of your own body and how to best care for it, as a helping hand along the way.

# ABOUT THE AUTHOR

Dr Nighat Arif is a GP specialising in women's health and family planning with over 16 years experience in the NHS and private practice. She is based in Buckinghamshire and is able to consult fluently with patients in Urdu and Punjabi. Dr Nighat is a medical educator and provides teaching to local trainee GPs as well as at national and international conferences. Dr Nighat was nominated for the National Bevan Prize for Health and Wellbeing to acknowledge her exceptional commitment to advancing wellbeing in her community. Dr Nighat has worked to raise awareness on menopause and women's healthcare in Black and Asian women, she presented her clinical work at the 'Menopause in the Workplace' Parliamentary committee hearing. She has also worked with Team Halo, a United Nation (UN) initiative to bring an end to the pandemic and presented at the G7 Global Vaccine Confidence Summit that led to her being awarded an Honorary Doctorate Degree in Science at London City University for Women's Health, Public Health and Inclusion. She is the honorary recipient of the 2023 SHE Award and received a Points of Light Award 2023 from the UK Prime Minister in recognition of her exceptional service to raising awareness for women's health in the UK.

Dr Nighat is the resident doctor on *BBC Breakfast*, ITV'S *This Morning* and BBC *LookEast*, and she hosts her own Sunday Breakfast show on BBC3 Counties Radio. Dr Nighat was also a contributor on the Channel 4 documentary *Davina McCall: Sex, Lies and the Menopause* and has made guest appearances on numerous podcasts tackling taboos around women's health. Dr Nighat has regularly written for various publications including *Stylist*, *HELLO*, *Red*, *Good Housekeeping* and *Women in Medicine* and her work around menopause has featured in *British Vogue*. She is also the ambassador of a global charity Wellbeing of Women, Roald Dahl's Marvellous Children's Charity, The Good Grief Trust, HerSpirit, Sikh Forgiveness and Upon Noon. She lives in Buckinghamshire with her husband and three sons.

@DrNighatArif

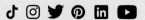

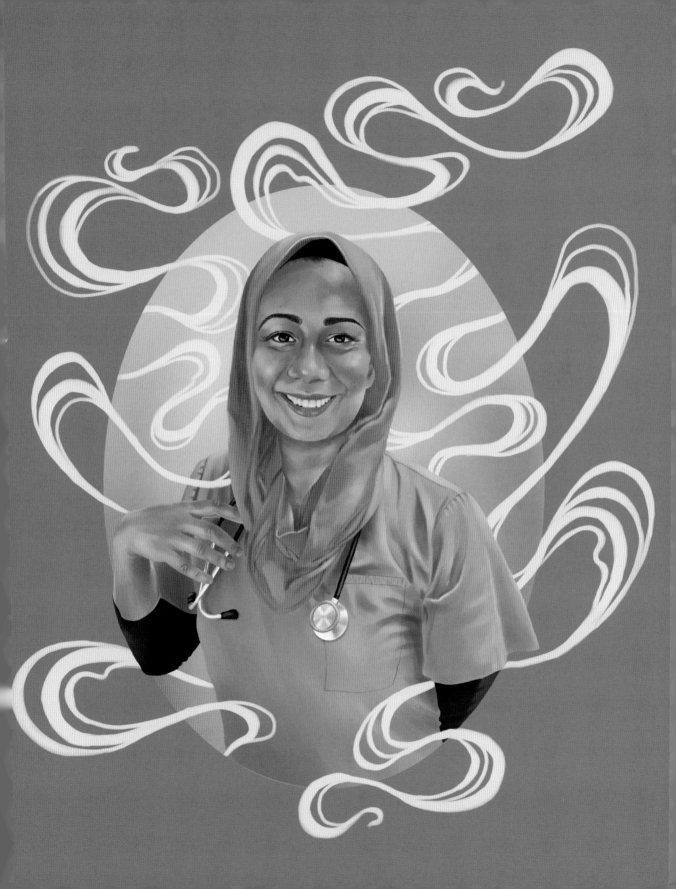

# ASTER*

First published in Great Britain in 2023 by Aster,
an imprint of
Octopus Publishing Group Ltd
Carmelite House
50 Victoria Embankment
London EC4Y 0DZ
www.octopusbooks.co.uk

An Hachette UK Company
www.hachette.co.uk

The authorized representative in the EEA is Hachette
Ireland, 8 Castlecourt Centre, Dublin 15, D15 XTP3, Ireland
(email: info@hbgi.ie)

ISBN 978-1-78325-523-8

A CIP catalogue record for this book is available
from the British Library.

Printed and bound in China

10 9 8 7 6 5 4 3 2

Publisher: Stephanie Jackson
Senior Editor: Pauline Bache
Art Director: Jaz Bahra
Words Contributor: Joanne Lake
Illustrator: Liliana Rasmussen
Picture Research: Giulia Hetherington and Jennifer Veall
Copy Editor: Joanne Smith
Assistant Production Manager: Emily Noto

Before making any changes in your health regime,
or starting any medical treatment, always consult
your own doctor for advice relevant to your
individual circumstances.

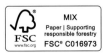